"In a book as warm and reassuring as a country doctor on a house call, Ruth McGinnis has not only given us a practical guide to healthy living, but shown us that getting—and keeping—fit doesn't have to take a lot of time or cost a lot of money. This is exactly what America needs to hear."

BILL FRIST, M.D., U.S. SENATOR (R-TENNESSEE)

"Ruth McGinnis maintains that for people to be healthy they must become well-rounded individuals, incorporating diet, exercise, and rest into the health equation. She even deals with such lifestyle issues as the intrusion of television and its time-robbing effect upon our lives. Thoughtfully written, *Living the Good Life* is a pleasure to read and will appeal primarily to women, but the simple principles are universally applicable."

CHRISTIAN RETAILING MAGAZINE

"With so many health-conscious books on the shelves these days it's refreshing to find one that really stands out from the crowd. Ruth McGinnis . . . offers a sensible approach to living a full, healthy life, taking things one step further by exploring the spiritual and emotional balances. This book is perfect for anyone seeking an all-encompassing, healthy lifestyle, and who enjoys a great read."

NASHVILLE PARENTS MAGAZINE

"Ruth McGinnis makes a compelling case not just for a healthier lifestyle, but for a life with meaning. Her approach to wellness is spiritually uplifting and leaves the reader with a sense of hope."

DR. ROBERT SCHULLER
PASTOR OF *THE HOUR OF POWER* AND THE CRYSTAL CATHEDRAL

"Ruth McGinnis' *Living the Good Life* is a wonderful book that offers sound advice on achieving inner and outer beauty without using trendy diets, fad fitness, or empty self-help theories. Her approach gives us hope that we can achieve peace and balance in our hectic schedules. Stop and smell the roses with Ruth, and learn how to enjoy the very good life our Creator has given us."

SHELLEY BREEN, POINT OF GRACE

D1258696

Total Health for Body & Soul

Ruth McGinnis

Foreword by Amy Grant

SPIRE

© 1998, 2001 by Ruth McGinnis

Published by Fleming H. Revell
a division of Baker Publishing Group
P.O. Box 6287, Grand Rapids, MI 49516-6287
www.revellbooks.com

Spire edition published 2005
ISBN 0-8007-8723-4

Revised edition of *The Good Life*, Thomas Nelson, Inc. Published by Fleming H. Revell in 2001 as *Living the Good Life*.

Printed in the United States of America

The information in this book is solely for educational and motivational purposes and is not medical advice. Please consult a medical or health professional before starting any exercise, nutrition, or wellness program. The reader assumes all risks for performing the exercises and following the nutritional advice described in *Total Health for Body & Soul*.

Except in cases where specific permission was granted, the stories recorded in this book are composite descriptions of many individuals and settings. Any resemblance to persons living or dead is purely accidental.

To the memory of my beloved Aunt Cathy—

Catherine Fallon McGinnis England

———∞∞∞———

Contents

7

Acknowledgments

I am so grateful for the many people in my life who have supported and encouraged my creative efforts over the years, including the writing (and rewriting) of this book. I am especially thankful that Baker Book House has given me the opportunity to revisit my first manuscript, and experience its second incarnation.

I want to acknowledge some of the wonderful people who have contributed to *Total Health for Body & Soul:*

- Randy Piland for pursuing a human interest story that led to my first publishing deal.
- Janet Thoma for her special role in my literary career.
- Gary Glover for his friendship and counsel.
- David Dunham for his friendship, loyalty, and literary representation.
- Jeanette Thomason for her beautiful editorial direction the second time around.
- My aunts Lois Huber, Crystalle Davis, and my mother, Freddie Lu Huber McGinnis, who were invaluable resources as I researched the lives of Grandma and Grandpa Huber.
- My aunt Marian Hurley, who scoured my first drafts with love and an English professor's relentless corrections.
- Dereama Sherrill for her role as Girl Friday in my hectic moments.
- Drs. Ann Evers and Gary Smith; physical therapist Tom Purvis;

counselors Shirley Jaeger, Bedford Combs, and Susan Crumpton; and Judi Adams, president of the Wheat Foods Council, for their much appreciated professional feedback.
- Pastors Jim Bachmann and Ian Sears for their spiritual support and guidance.

I must also thank the clients and workshop participants I've been privileged to meet and work with over the years, who have influenced me more than they can ever imagine. I've learned so much by being part of their amazing processes of change.

Amy, thank you for these many years of friendship and the unique professional opportunities you have so generously shared. (And for visiting your eloquent foreword a second time.)

I'm also grateful for my family; my parents Frank and Freddie Lu McGinnis, and sisters, Julie, Laura, Rachel, and Erin, for loving me throughout life's twisting path.

Finally, I thank my husband, John Burrell, who has encouraged my creative efforts over the years with enthusiasm, patience, and financial support.

Foreword

I first met Ruth in February of 1993, four months after the birth of my third child, Sarah. As any new mother will tell you, during this nursing-intensive stretch of life, one's emotional pendulum can swing pretty hard from euphoria to despair. Sleepless nights, the constant demands of motherhood, and an unrecognizable body shape had me feeling overwhelmed. In spite of the positive pressure to get in shape that work has provided me over the years, I couldn't seem to muster the enthusiasm to invest in my physical appearance this third time around. What did sound good to me was cashing in my collection of 501 Levis and investing in an affordable line of muumuus.

Enter Ruth.

On the recommendation of a long time friend in the music business, who had some real results working with Ruth, I made an appointment. I had a very exercise-intensive, body-buffing daily regime with a trainer several years ago; even though the contoured physique staring back at me in the mirror was one I never thought I would see, I still came away from that time feeling pressured and inadequate to maintain yet another area of my life.

How can I put into words the impact of the journey that I began that day with Ruth? We started at the beginning . . . with balance, posture, and simple exercises that she explained would build up my infrastructure—the subtle strength around the joints that protects your body. She encouraged me to walk or jog or do anything to get my metabolism going. I didn't. I couldn't yet.

Still, she would show up at my house, and week by week we would work on the same principles: balance, subtle structural strength, and gradually we added small increments of weight. And we talked. We talked about what a healthy mental image for a woman in her thirties would be, and how that differs from a healthy image of a twenty-year-old, a sixty-year-old, etc. We talked about family, about relationships, about life.

In a way I was envious of Ruth for the simplicity of her life. She had no children, a job where she called her own shots, fewer demands on her time. She celebrated simple things that I wanted to celebrate but was too busy to enjoy. Over time, I began to see Ruth's life more clearly . . . her unique pressures, the demands on her heart, her mind, and her time. I relearned the lesson that no one has the perfect scenario. We are all invested in other people, in work, in dreams for the future, and so we all experience the same kinds of pressures in life.

Slowly, something began to change me. Almost a year into my work with Ruth, I went on my first jog. I started making time to walk. What I was compelled by in Ruth was a centeredness in her spirit, an absence of any manipulation of me, but a genuine desire in her for me to value and cherish the life that had been given to me by God.

In exploring my motivations for exercise, I was forced to take a long, hard look at the way I valued my own life, not for what I was able to do for others, not for what I brought to my family, not for what anyone else thought of me, but what value did I place on my own existence, on my own journey through life?

As I started to experience a change in attitude toward my own body, I began to feel continental shifts in other areas of my life. How could I honor my body and yet turn a blind eye to emotional areas of my life where I was so embroiled in denial and pain that I was merely functioning? Ruth had warned me that I couldn't look at changing one part of my life without being willing to change other areas. Of course, I didn't understand what she meant at the time. Now I do.

Along the road to my own health, Ruth has given me books to read. We joke about the fact that I have skimmed them all and finished none. But the process is underway. The simple exercises that Ruth and I have been doing for years, the exercise of respect toward myself and others, the exercise of taking a simpler approach to life have strengthened not only my body but my mind and spirit as well.

When Ruth told me that she was going to write a book about her approach to health, I was thrilled. I just hoped that she could capture the simple essence of her example in words. I respect Ruth as a musician, a health and fitness professional, a woman, a friend, and now a writer. She has been more of an inspiration to me than she could ever know.

This book is a celebration of the sacred journey of life. Simple. Profound.

What a pleasure it is to be adding a post script to the foreword that I wrote for Ruth's book back in 1997. I'm happy to report that we are once again in the process of unearthing my post-partum body, following the joyful arrival of my fourth child, Corrina Grant Gill.

The integrity of Ruth's approach to health and fitness has stood the test of time for me, and the journey continues to be worth every step.

One

A Return
to Simple Principles

She girds herself with strength,
And strengthens her arms.
Strength and honor are her clothing;
she shall rejoice in time to come.

PROVERBS 31:17, 25 (NKJV)

My Grandpa Huber was a farmer for most of his life in Menomonie, Wisconsin. He labored hard, as many did in that era, making a living by the sweat of his brow. He rose before the sun came up and went to bed after the sun went down.

He and Grandmother kept an enormous garden filled with every imaginable fruit and vegetable that would grow in that northern climate. Their watermelons were so good, they had to be hidden in the corn rows or risk being "cooned."

My grandmother canned and preserved throughout the growing season, and that single garden provided most of my grandparents' food all year round. Grandma started baking early in the morning, and by breakfast time had loaves in the oven and hot, fragrant biscuits on the table. Meat and dairy products also came fresh from the farm; the only supplies my grandmother bought from the grocery store were flour, sugar, and salt.

Every day after lunch, Grandfather sat down in his rocking chair for a half-hour nap before returning to the fields. Evenings tended to be quiet—a good time for conversation, reading, or a game of checkers.

My grandparents rose early, worked hard, ate wholesome foods, and got plenty of sleep. They also honored Sunday as a day of rest. Grandpa would let hay rot in the fields rather than labor on the Sabbath. The tapestry of their rustic life was woven with devotion to family, faith, and working the land.

This simple lifestyle illustrates something I've long suspected—that human beings are equipped with enormous potential to live the good life. The lovely, down-to-earth rhythm my grandparents experienced was consistent with the way people had lived for centuries. Life wasn't easy, but it was less complicated than what we know today: People didn't worry about getting enough exercise, since physical activity was built into their daily rounds. Food wasn't an issue unless it was scarce, and it tended to be unrefined and healthy. Folks didn't worry about weapons of mass destruction, global warming, or guns in school. Terms like "multi-tasking," "24-7," and "burnout" hadn't been invented. But perhaps the most striking characteristic of my grandparents' time was the absence of the intense need most of us feel for amazing personal achievement, acquiring material things, and looking perfect on the outside.

Today, as we routinely deal with stresses never before known to the human race, including the enormous pressure we put on ourselves, it's no wonder we struggle to attain even a small measure of well-being and satisfaction in life.

I became acquainted with this struggle my first year in college. Armed with the unrealistic dream of becoming a concert violinist, a dream I'd fostered since the age of eight, I walked into my freshman year with a long list of self-imposed expectations. I tried to adhere to my well-laid plans, which included carrying a double major in music and English, practicing three hours a day, improving my complexion, and attracting the perfect husband. But I began to bump into my human limitations. My tendency to eat for emotional comfort, something that started in high school, was catching up with me. In addition to almost never managing to get in that three hours of daily practice, my skin was getting worse, and I was putting on unwanted weight. By the end of my freshmen year, I'd gained nearly thirty pounds and was miserable with myself.

This difficult period coincided with the early days of the fitness revolution of the 1970s. The first Jane Fonda workout videos had hit the marketplace, running had become a national pastime, and every women's magazine had the latest diet promising quick and easy weight loss or the best exercises to get thin thighs and a flat stomach.

Intrigued by the beautiful bodies that promoted the fitness craze, I decided to start running as a way to lose weight. The day I put on a pair of running shoes marked the beginning of a lifelong love of being physically active. It also made for another achievement to add to my list: physical perfection.

In an ensuing ten-year obsession to be model-thin, I would try all kinds of diets, fasting, and frequently take exercise to unhealthy extremes. By the time I reached Juilliard, where I finished my music degrees, I was weighing myself three times a day. But no matter what the scale said or how well I was doing at school, it never seemed to be good enough.

Today I feel unspeakable sadness for the perfectly appointed life I tried for so long to attain, at the cost of wasted years and life experiences. Yet I also feel the exhilaration of being free of my relentless expectations, and gratitude for having the chance to live my life differently. Perhaps you're reading these words and feeling the weight of your own expectations and disappointments in life. If so, I encourage you to consider the possibility that you too can experience a different kind of life.

Mine started to change after graduating from Juilliard. While floundering for career direction in New York, I'd become intrigued with the freedom and beauty of other styles of music, including folk, country, and bluegrass fiddle. So I moved to Nashville in 1986 to pursue this new genre, and stumbled into a new career interest—health and wellness. I signed up for classes at a Nashville fitness studio, concerned as always about my exercise regimen. But, fortunately, and I think not accidentally, this studio was years ahead of its time, touting a philosophy of wellness more than the pursuit of body parts of steel.

In this positive environment, I became interested in being certified as an instructor. As I learned more about the complex nature of the whole person, I grappled with my misguided zeal for a perfect-looking body. In order to teach others balanced exercise routines and the importance of good nutrition and rest, I knew I had to resolve my own unhealthy habits and body image issues. I embarked on a humbling and sometimes painful process of emotional and spiritual healing, and discovered along the way what I had to offer as a wellness professional.

Gradually I found myself less drawn to the extreme mantras of the fitness revolution and more interested in the big picture of being healthy and well. I became certified as a personal trainer and wellness advisor so I could take on a more meaningful role in people's lives. As I worked closely with others, especially women, in the quest for a better life, I was struck with the universal nature of this challenge. Every person wants to live the best life possible. Every person wants to be physically and emotionally strong, know a measure of balance every day, and develop their potential for beauty. Despite best efforts, however, these desires too often become just another burden to bear, another agenda to never get right, another disappointing and elusive dream.

I'd love to tell you that by reading this book you'll be able to break through all your failures and disappointments, and that you'll finally live the good life you always dreamed possible. But I can't.

I can tell you, though, as someone who has dreamed, failed miserably, and lived to dream again, that you can discover a different way of looking at things, a new understanding of the basics of taking care of the self, and new tools for making life-enhancing choices.

This different perspective on self and health improvement begins with three important principles.

The first is the concept of the whole person: Whatever changes you hope to make in any area of your life must respect and integrate the physical, emotional, and spiritual components within. It's futile to embrace the discipline of exercise and good nutrition without addressing the emotional and spiritual issues that might thwart your efforts. After all, your physical body (experienced through your five senses) is intrinsically intertwined with your emotional blueprint (affecting feelings, reasoning, and behavior), and with your spirit (which yearns to connect with eternity). This fascinatingly complex package shows up everywhere you go and in everything you do.

The second principle is the challenge of our times: Your precious, unique, whole person is bombarded daily with unprecedented cultural change. The simpler life my grandparents knew is no more; people are ill-equipped to handle the combined stresses absorbed daily from our culture's environment, media, and breathtaking pace in every area of life. While understanding the challenge of these times will not return anyone to a simpler existence, it can put a name to what we're up against. Also recognizing this challenge is the first step toward dealing with it.

Finally there's the principle of the power of choice: Every day you make small choices that add up over a lifetime to powerfully affect your wellbeing. Yet how often do you feel helpless about all the things that affect your life over which you have no control? How many times, when starting a new regimen, do you fall for the myth that you have to do something huge, expensive, or time-consuming in order to make a difference? Most folks today could transform their quality of life by simply choosing to get a little more sleep each night and drinking two liters of water every day. Instead of berating yourself for the things you never accomplish, you can acknowledge the value of the small things you do.

So what is the good life? While there's no single definition, and certainly no wrong one, it involves a basic foundation. It requires a childlike joy and fascination for the minutia of life: The ability to appreciate the smell of coffee brewing first thing in the morning, or the miracle of a puppy's soft, sweet face, or the awesome splendor of the sky at sunset.

The good life is something we're more likely to experience with a sense of physical, emotional, and spiritual well-being. It helps to have a sense of financial peace by living within our means. It includes feeling involved in something beyond our own happiness and understanding the value of all life. And it's perpetually changing—the good life desired at midlife will be different from what you dreamed of in your twenties, which is as it should be.

So I invite you on this journey toward living a better life. Bring your personal hopes and dreams, whatever they may be, and prepare to explore the multifaceted elements of personal change—including motivation, exercise, nutrition, balance, self-responsibility, and spiritual and emotional health. As you do so, your dreams will come into clearer focus.

The strength, balance, and beauty you seek in yourself and in life, are part of a quest as old as time. It's an honorable one. My grandparents sought it in their time, and our children will seek it also.

Two

Motivation

*If one advances confidently in the
direction of his dreams, and endeavors
to live the life which he has imagined,
he will meet with a success unexpected
in common hours.*

HENRY DAVID THOREAU

Every January, after the food fest of the holidays has run its course, fitness clubs and diet centers are flooded with customers newly motivated to lose weight and get in shape. Teaching in an exercise studio, I witnessed this phenomenon year after year. We sold more memberships during the first week of January than any other time of the year, and classes were filled to capacity every hour of the day.

By February, however, membership sales and class sizes returned to normal. The burst of enthusiasm fueled by New Year's resolutions, like many types of motivation, has limited staying power in the face of the challenging process of change. Regardless of how committed we are to self-improvement, the way we motivate ourselves inevitably influences our quest for a healthier lifestyle.

As a wellness professional I'm constantly aware of the important role motivation plays in making positive lifestyle changes. Early in my career, a client drove this point home in a way I'll never forget. A lady called, inquiring about my services. She wanted to get together right away, so I drove to her home in a wealthy section of Nashville and was ushered inside by the maid.

I admit I was excited about the potential of this client because she could afford my services, had the time to work out regularly, and seemed a good prospect for referrals.

Then Cassandra entered the room where I was waiting with my health questionnaire and training bag. She was in her forties, an attractive woman with blonde hair, carrying an extra twenty pounds on her 5'5" frame. She seemed preoccupied and a little nervous. I tried to soothe her nerves and began the consultation by asking about her health history and general lifestyle, what she hoped to achieve through her workouts, and when we could schedule a regular time to meet.

Cassandra jumped up and ran into the bedroom, returning with a cocktail dress two sizes too small. "I need to get into this dress in time for my Christmas party," she declared. "That's why I called you."

I sat across the room on her expensive couch, my heart sinking. Cassandra continued her litany of reasons for needing to lose weight: She had eaten too much over Thanksgiving. Her husband was dropping hints about her appearance. Her best friend had just crash-dieted off ten pounds and looked great. On and on she went with desperation in her voice.

Quietly I listened, knowing there was no healthy way to get her into that dress in three weeks' time. I thought of the inherent challenge we face in achieving a healthy lifestyle and remembered how rough my own path had been.

Like Cassandra, I used to measure my happiness and self-worth by a dress size. Like her friend and many others, I'd tried all kinds of crash diets to drop a quick ten pounds. But it wasn't to be healthier. It was because I wanted to look like model Cheryl Tiegs. I wanted a sexy, beautiful body—and I wanted it as quickly as possible.

Twenty-five years later I'm still exercising, but for a much different reason. I've let go of unrealistic goals of fitness, and my concept of a beautiful body has changed too. I've learned to be honest and more gentle with myself, finally admitting that excessive exercise and obsessive eating habits are not healthy. I stopped measuring my self-worth by a number on the scale and eventually even stopped getting on the scale. As my motivation changed my approach to health shifted to something I could live with, which has resulted in more consistency and inner peace.

‒‒‒‒‒‒

I know if I do it just one more time, I can get it right.
ANONYMOUS

Still, I recognize how many other women identify with Cassandra's story, and my own. Who hasn't started a diet and exercise program only to fizzle out after a few weeks? Who isn't eager to see changes in the mirror and on the scale, but when these changes don't happen on schedule, feels waning enthusiasm? These are classic reactions when unrealistic goals are set for yourself and your body, or when the primary motivation to exercise or eat right is based on a quick cosmetic return. Bursts of inspiration to change one's looks won't get anyone very far, however, because there's not enough substance behind the commitment.

My job as a fitness trainer and wellness professional is to help people make lifestyle changes that last. Toward that end, I encourage health as the primary motivation for the efforts. Any lifestyle change takes hard work and an investment of time, and the visible results won't happen overnight. You can buy equipment, learn exercise routines, join the health club, and invest in a diet plan—but none of these things will make a difference if you don't move from desire to action. Motivation is that all-important step. When you're consistently motivated to take good care of your body, with the big picture and the long term firmly in mind, you'll have success.

My greatest joy is witnessing the success of a client who has chosen the road to health for all the right reasons. This generally happens after a few false starts followed by a period of frustration and regrouping. It's perfectly normal to set a goal, experience a brief period of successful follow-through, then have everything fall apart. In fact this happens every New Year, when masses make resolutions for better health that are recanted by February.

Why? You can attribute this tendency to two major obstacles. One is the daily battle we all wage with human nature. The other is the image of physical perfection that's become a cultural standard for the pursuit of health and fitness, a challenge of our time. Overcoming these obstacles isn't easy, but understanding them is a big step toward developing the sort of motivation that will last a lifetime.

—⁂—

O LORD, you have searched me and you know me . . .
you are familiar with all my ways.

PSALM 139:1, 3

As human beings we're faced daily with personal shortcomings and weaknesses. Human nature encourages us to take the path of least resistance, and do what we want rather than what we ought. It's much easier, for example, to fall on the couch in front of the TV at the end of a long day rather than head out the door for a brisk thirty-minute walk. Eating rich, high-calorie foods is usually more appealing than munching on raw fruits and vegetables. Settling for the cool decay of a relationship that's not working is far easier than getting professional counseling to work toward resolution.

These are all examples of human nature at work—and believe me, I'm no stranger to any of them. That's why I love a statement of truth that M. Scott Peck makes at the beginning of his classic *The Road Less Traveled:* "Life is difficult." Those three words sum up beautifully the inherent struggle in life and apply perfectly to the process of positive change.

I've experienced the reality of this myself and with every person I've worked with. A client will inevitably get frustrated with the process and say, "I meant to get on the bike every night after work this week, and I just didn't do it." Or, if the issue is food-related, I hear, "Every day I do great until 3:00 P.M., but then I start snacking, and before long I've completely blown my food plan."

I respond: "Staying on a healthy regimen for life is one of the hardest things you'll ever do. It's a lifelong endeavor, a road with twists and turns, many challenges, and setbacks. But it's achievable and worth every effort you make."

I never know exactly when I'll get to this point with a client, but when it comes, it's a wonderful breakthrough. The client understands that healthy living is an ongoing process. The path takes on more importance than the destination, and in this way it can be a gift to bump up against our human nature and acknowledge our limitations.

As Peck says, "Once we know that life is difficult—once we truly understand and accept it—then life is no longer difficult."

This principle can be applied to the pursuit of wellness. Once you accept the fact that a disciplined lifestyle is a difficult process, it becomes less hard—regardless of whether the issue is choosing

25

activity over laziness, eating a prudent diet, or committing to emotional and spiritual growth.

———

Do not deceive yourselves. If any one of you thinks he is wise by the standards of this age, he should become a "fool" so that he may become wise. For the wisdom of this world is foolishness in God's sight.

1 CORINTHIANS 3:18–19

The other big challenge on the course for positive change is staying focused on true healthy living. It's easy to be misled by media images that permeate our cultural understanding of health and fitness. Pick up any popular women's or fitness magazine and you'll see what I mean. There's always an article about the diet secrets of a Hollywood star or exercises a big celebrity does with her star trainer. Fashion pages are filled with clothes most women couldn't wear, on the gaunt bodies that most women don't have. The advertising industry sets a glossy standard of physical perfection that the majority of people cannot attain, a standard that ultimately has little to do with being healthy and living well.

I know how alluring these images can be. I tried to emulate them for years, even at the risk of my personal health. While dwelling on these images or using them as a measuring stick for success is understandable, it ultimately leads to frustration.

A beautiful model might be nice to look at, but what does anyone know about her life? She might smoke, abuse alcohol or drugs, and suffer from an eating disorder—something rampant in the modeling industry. Is she healthy or happy? Does she eat a good diet or exercise regularly? Does she feel strong? Can physical attractiveness ever automatically mean wellness, happiness, or purposefulness?

Television and film try to answer such questions with mixed messages. I can't count the number of "fitness" features I've seen on shows like *Entertainment Tonight* profiling healthy role models who obviously had plastic surgery to enhance their physiques. These personalities promote the latest exercise video or demonstrate how they stay looking good for a nude scene in some current movie. Their bodies are lean, but curvy in all the right places. Their faces are unlined but tanned. They show us how easy it is to be beautiful, but there's a great irony at work here.

More often than not, these personalities have gone to the tanning bed and the surgeon to help achieve that perfect look. Tanning, of course, ages the skin and is a leading cause of skin cancer; plastic surgery can have side effects. No one really knows yet the long-term health implications of breast implants, liposuction, and other cosmetic procedures. While I have no personal objection with surgery being available to those who choose it, I do think it's unfair to hold up surgically altered bodies as a standard of beauty or fitness. The taut, tanned, curvy-but-dimpleless body is a constant presence in the marketing of health, fitness, and beauty. Yet comparing ourselves to such images of unattainable perfection is destructive.

Another phenomenon confusing the issue of health are the diet and exercise infomercials, or paid programming, that run almost constantly on cable TV. Celebrities and fitness industry stars promote every imaginable gadget or machine to solve—once and for all—anyone's weight and figure problems. The formula is basically the same regardless of personality or product. It strikes a nerve with human behavior, and people from all walks of life will plunk down three easy payments of $29.95 for one piece of equipment after another. The message is clever and simple: "Buy this product and you will quickly and easily transform your lumpy body into a vision of healthful loveliness in just a few short weeks."

I've had some personal experiences with these infomercial gadgets. A few years ago, I was working out with two women who owned a house and a business together and were making a joint effort to get on a fitness program. I've rarely enjoyed clients more than this bright, hardworking, churchgoing, attractive, fun duo. One day I walked into our workout area and saw a plastic contraption that looked like a child's toy, a gray-and-orange thing shaped like a rocket, on the floor. It was one of the current abdominal exercisers being promoted on television, and it gave me a good dose of insight, once again, into human nature.

My bright, articulate, well-educated clients had been enticed by persuasive marketing to buy something they didn't need. Who wouldn't want a piece of equipment to provide motivation, muscles, and instant results? But only in the cunning script of the marketing beast could that happen.

The fact is, no one can buy motivation, and no one needs to spend money on things to become healthier and more attractive. External forces will always be present to make people think otherwise, but deep down inside the truth can be known: Health is something no one can buy.

<hr />

*Dear friend, I pray that you may enjoy good health
and that all may go well with you . . .*
3 JOHN 1:2

As you wake every morning, you have an opportunity to embrace the day with choices that are good for you. Over the course of a day there will be many things you can't control, but your health is something you can positively affect.

I know that if I accomplish nothing else of value, I can exercise my power of choice: drink plenty of water, eat numerous servings of fruits and vegetables, accumulate thirty minutes of activity in the span of my day—and be better for all of it. I make these healthy choices as often as I can because I want to live long and live well. I want to enjoy whatever time I have on this earth in a body that's pain-free, functional, and energetic.

At times, though, your body can become an issue. This is especially true on the day you miss the rich experience of life because you're sick, tired, depressed, injured, or so distracted by your appearance that you don't want to leave the house.

Times like that in my life fill me with regret today because I can never have those years back to live differently—and how much of life I missed. During my first year in college, when I gained nearly thirty pounds, I struggled with unrealistic expectations of myself as an

28

aspiring violinist and college student. There weren't enough hours in the day to do all I felt I needed in order to be as accomplished as I should be, so I turned to eating as a means of comfort and distraction and a way to medicate my emotional pain.

The weight gain was just the beginning of a downward spiral. As I became uncomfortable with my body and ashamed of my appearance, I tended to isolate myself and, of course, eat more. Then I started beating myself up with strenuous diets, fasting, and compulsive exercise. This behavior was as much a prison as the food addiction. I held myself back from all kinds of experiences because I wasn't eating that week or hadn't done the two-hour advanced Jane Fonda workout that day.

I learned how my body could be an issue in another way too—about fifteen years ago, when years of fiddle playing caught up with my upper back. I began to experience debilitating muscle spasms that left me in tears and frustration. These episodes took on a pattern: Long hours of nonstop fiddle playing, combined with physical exhaustion and stress, resulted in back traumas that lasted up to a week. I learned what injury and pain could do to my well-planned life at a moment's notice.

It took several episodes of painful bouts before I finally found the solution: self-care. I started a strength-training routine for my back, booked regular massage-therapy sessions, and established a relationship with a good chiropractor. I've enjoyed living in a pain-free body ever since. Having experienced my body as an issue, and knowing it doesn't have to be that way, keeps me motivated to take care of myself and to embrace a healthy lifestyle.

Most of us don't consider the value of good health until it's threatened. It's human nature to take the body and physical abilities for granted, then from time to time a wake-up call comes as a reminder that health is invaluable and worth making a priority. Who hasn't experienced aches and pains, illness and injury? These wake-up calls need to be treated with respect. Just as bumping into some road block, set up to keep you from going over a cliff, can be a gift, so can a bout with pain and illness. These things serve as a reminder of what really matters on a daily basis, and can be a catalyst for doing things necessary to reclaim health.

A music producer I worked with a few years ago experienced this phenomenon. Brown suffered from terrible migraine headaches, and when these headaches hit, his entire life was thrown into chaos. Record projects would grind to a halt, his family had to tiptoe around him, and he missed a lot of sweet moments in life because he was at the mercy of those headaches. Through spurts of exercise and sporadic lifestyle adjustments he found some relief, but it was inconsistent. One day his headache was so debilitating, he had to go to the emergency room for treatment. But his body was so used to pain medication, he had to be anesthetized to experience relief from the excruciating pain.

The day Brown left the hospital he promised to make his health top priority. He threw out all his pain killers, muscled through the withdrawal headaches, and went on a caffeine-, sugar-, and dairy-free diet. He's been faithful to his new regimen, which also includes regular sleep hours and exercise sessions, for more than a year and no longer gets headaches.

See how a negative situation, like recurring headaches, can be turned into motivation for changing a lifestyle? And see how not just the person doing the changing, but family, friends, and work all benefit from such positive change? The body is no longer an issue.

The desire to reclaim and maintain wellness is the seed of motivation that makes the difference between a temporary fix and a long-term solution. Your body is a gift from God and you can take care of it. When you can gratefully acknowledge what a gift it is to feel good, to be able to function, to actively enjoy life, you'll find the motivation to be healthy for life.

I love witnessing people's success with this mind-set in place. They do their best to adhere to their programs—and whenever they feel tripped up by inevitable lapses, they keep coming back to the basics. They remind themselves not to get bogged down with dress sizes, body fat measurements, or numbers on a scale. They return to the thinking that helped them choose wellness not as an option, but a priority. They embrace their pursuit of health as a process and make the commitment to it for life.

Ironically, the subjects of these success stories are also the ones who enjoy not only pounds and inches lost, but the cosmetic benefits of self-care. They tend to enjoy a better quality of life, follow through on their wellness commitments, and achieve the best results too.

As for Cassandra, I never did get a program together with her. I knew, sadly, I couldn't help her lose the two dress sizes she desired in three weeks. But our encounter was not without some benefit; in this case, the trainer learned more from the client. Cassandra reminded me how much baggage, misunderstanding, and illusion there is to cut through to make meaningful life changes.

So if Cassandra, or you, came to me today, eager to exercise and bearing a cocktail dress as a measuring stick, this is what I would say: "Stop beating yourself up with a dress that's too small for you. Instead, prepare yourself for a long and fascinating process of change. Let the outward changes, the inches lost or muscles toned, be the icing on the cake. Focus on the changes you feel more keenly than the changes you see. Try to embrace the journey rather than the destination."

There will never be that magical place where you've made it, gotten it, or attained the perfect-looking body. That's a myth of our culture. The pursuit of health is continuous, a long series of efforts that span a lifetime. With each effort you'll be rewarded with a sense of well-being that can help fuel the next effort. And every step you take—whether it's drinking eight glasses of water a day or fitting a ten-minute walk into your schedule, mastering the push-up or taking time to be quiet—is a step forward.

Celebrate each step.

One day you'll wake up and notice that your back doesn't hurt, or that you've made it through the winter without getting a cold, or that your stamina has increased, and you'll feel like doing more with your family. This is the moment to revel. The potential to live a healthy life is always inside of you waiting to be born.

The Power of Choice

Things you can do every day to impact your well-being

- **Record your progress toward healthy living in a small notebook.** This is your daily wellness journal, where you'll keep track of things like how much water you consume, fruit you eat, and exercise you've done. This can be as simple or involved as you want.

- **Think of the person you want to be in 10, 30, or 50 years.** Picture the energy, physical ability, and productivity you want. Think of the gift you'd give yourself and others by taking care of yourself today.

- **Know the facts about how small efforts add up to your benefit.** There's substantial evidence that even thirty minutes of moderate activity accumulated over the course of one day, every day, can significantly reduce the risk of heart disease, strokes, and some cancers.

- **Focus on the gratitude you have after an illness.** You know the day you really start feeling better after a bad cold has passed? How easy it is to forget that sense of gratitude and sweet relief for just feeling better. Say a prayer of thanks for what you have today, and resolve to do something good for your body.

- **Give yourself permission to start over with your exercise, food plan, and spiritual growth as often as you like.** Nothing is more defeating than an all-or-nothing attitude. Remind yourself: "I may renegotiate my goals—any and all good intentions—as often as necessary. I can start over as many times as I need to or want."

Three

Exercise
Back-to-Basics

Ex-er-cise . . . 3. activity for training
or developing the body or mind; esp.,
bodily exertion for the sake of health.

WEBSTER'S NEW WORLD DICTIONARY

What does the word "exercise" mean to you? Does it conjure up something positive or negative? The fact is, exercise is written about and talked about so frequently, it's impossible not to have some personal connotation of it. For some that connotation is negative: blood, sweat, tears, failure. For others it means time and effort well spent, stress relief for the body and mind, a means to control weight.

Since only a fraction of the adults in our country exercise on a regular basis, it seems more people identify with the first definition than the second. This is a shame, because a reasonable amount of exercise done every day is like drinking from the fountain of youth, and I'm convinced everyone can find a way to include activity and movement in daily life.

I like Webster's definition of exercise, especially the phrase "bodily exertion for the sake of health." What a marvelous degree of latitude that gives; it can include virtually anything that involves physical effort or movement. To be a successful exerciser means allowing a great deal of flexibility in your programs. This happens when exercise is more than something done in a class or gym for thirty to sixty minutes several times a week.

One thing I've found helpful in creating good connotations for "exercise" is to remember people have exercised long before the fitness revolution taught us how important it was to our health or before Webster defined it as "bodily exertion." People have been exercising since the beginning of time.

My Grandpa and Grandma Huber would be stupefied by the lifestyles we lead today, especially in the way we approach fitting in an exercise program. By the time I was born in 1957, my grandparents were well into their seventies, and I'm sure neither one of them had ever seen, let alone been on, a treadmill. They would probably think we'd all taken leave of our senses, given the money and angst our generations spend on exercise. For my grandparents, exercise was a way of life, not so much a choice as a necessity, from early in the morning until the sun went down at night.

Grandpa was up by 4:30 or 5:00 almost every morning. First thing, he would head to the barn, feed and milk the cows, separate the milk, and feed the hogs and chickens—all before breakfast, which was at seven. After that, he'd be in the fields where he planted, raised, and harvested alfalfa, corn, and wheat. During the winter he harvested ice—fifty-pound chunks that he would cut from the frozen river, lift out with huge ice tongs, coat with sawdust, and store in the ice house. He was physically active, extremely so by our standards, all day, every day, most of his life.

Grandma's days were no less active. She was up every morning at the crack of dawn, kneading dough for the breads, biscuits, and pies that she baked daily. She'd be up and down the cellar stairs many times a day to store food or get a jar of preserves or canned food; one-third of the basement was used to store the canned fruits, vegetables, and meats that she put up all year long. In addition to all the food preparation and housekeeping, she sewed every stitch of clothing the family wore, made quilts, and knitted and crocheted. Think of the effort it took to wash, wring, dry, and iron a load of laundry in those days without the electronic appliances we take for granted.

It wasn't unusual for my grandma to help out in the fields, either. She'd work right alongside Grandpa, stacking hay and sheaves of corn into shocks. Even when my mother was an infant, Grandma Huber would keep working, tucking her napping baby under the shade of the corn shocks.

In the length of one day, both of my grandparents probably used more muscle and expended more sweat and energy than any one person now does in the course of one week. Then, at the end of the day, they would spend quiet time by fire and candlelight before turning in early for a sound and restful night's sleep.

35

Fast-forward to the twenty-first century. Even if your grandparents didn't live on a farm, it's likely they were naturally and regularly physically active, much more so than you or I. Today we may be busier, but we don't use our bodies as much. Our conveniences of modern living require little or no physical exertion: cars, vacuum cleaners, dishwashers, washer-dryers—we don't even have to get off the sofa to change channels on our television sets! Herein lies the dilemma (or one of them) of our generation. We're naturally inactive, where our grandparents would have been active, and we're paying for our inactivity with weight gain and a general lack of fitness. Is it any wonder that weight loss and exercise programs have become such a national obsession?

---

*How often—even before we began—have we declared
a task "impossible"? And how often have we construed
a picture of ourselves as being inadequate?*

PIERO FERRUCCI

Over the past forty years the number of overweight Americans has increased dramatically. Survey after survey shows obesity growing at an alarming rate in men, women, and even in children; in July 1996, the Surgeon General finally added inactivity as a risk factor for premature death and disability. Yet despite billions of dollars spent annually on fitness and diet products, we're not making a dent in this terrible trend. In fact, while the fitness revolution that began in 1960 has provided plenty of information and inspiration for making exercise part of our lives, less than 25 percent of us do so on a regular basis.

How do we bridge the gap between good intentions and the actual follow-through of more physical activity?

The first step is to change the way we think about exercise and increase more opportunities for daily bodily exertion. Our culture has narrowed the parameters of what "exercise" means, and "physical activity," as a descriptive term, covers a lot more territory than we imagine.

I encourage you to begin thinking generally rather than specifically. Experience exercise as broad, open, and unlimited. Put aside the headlines, magazine covers, or news reports of the latest findings on exercise. Also put aside past attempts at regimens you've let fall by the wayside or memories of unpleasant experiences like P.E. class in school. (Did you dread going to P.E. as much as me? It's all too easy for me to remember failing the president's fitness test year after year, especially the sit-ups, or remember dangling helplessly from the pull-up bar in junior high.) Take any images like this from your past and gently let them go. Embrace a more tolerant and all-encompassing approach to exercise. What's important is not your method or even the duration, but rather the simple fact you choose activity over inactivity.

In fact I've seen firsthand how the things done physically every day impact your life and health over time more than any routine or program that's been taken on for just a few weeks or months.

One of the best examples of lifestyle-based fitness I can think of is my friend and client Bob. As a stock analyst who works from seven in the morning to six in the evening, Bob's on the job Monday through Friday, with quite a bit of travel. Most of his day entails sitting: at a desk, before a computer, talking on the phone, and in meetings. Several years ago he called me for help with an exercise routine because of chronic back pain that stemmed from sitting so much after injuries from an automobile accident.

We've since worked together, sometimes once a week, sometimes twice, always to keep Bob on some kind of therapeutic and strength-building exercise regimen. While he's motivated to exercise for all the right reasons, and his investment in personal training sessions is a testament of his dedication to pain-free living, Bob's beset with a challenge that faces almost everyone: There aren't enough hours in his day to fit in a regular exercise session.

As a husband with two young children, Bob already gets up at 5:45 A.M. to be at the office by 7:00, so getting up earlier to exercise isn't realistic. Neither is breaking away from the office during lunch to change clothes, work out at the gym, shower, change back into street clothes, and get back to his desk in an hour.

By the time Bob gets home from work, it's 6:30 or 7:00 P.M., and his wife needs help with the kids while she gets dinner on the table. That makes hopping on the exercise bike for twenty minutes at the end of the workday a rare opportunity. After some limited family time over dinner, there's barely time to do anything except shuffle through work papers and get to bed for a few hours of sleep before the next work day begins.

Doesn't this time crunch sound familiar? It's commonplace in our modern culture and affects men and women of all ages and all backgrounds. We can know exercise is important and desire to be active and well, but the daily grind gets in the way of our good intentions.

Here's where stretching the mental parameters of what exercise is can make such a difference. After trying several plans to get Bob active between training sessions (including swimming at lunch and biking only ten minutes after work), I admitted, "Bob, your life is simply not conducive to a formal exercise routine."

We needed to find ways for him to be more active during the course of his workday; the solution turned out to be incredibly simple and effective. I'd asked Bob to describe his routines from home to work. As soon as he mentioned parking in the first-level parking garage and taking an elevator to the eleventh floor, I asked him, "How many flights of stairs would you be willing to try walking up every day when you get to work instead of getting on the elevator?"

He was willing to commit to climbing at least nine flights, then riding the elevator the rest of the way as this was the only access route to his office. Bob became so enthusiastic about this solution, he then volunteered to take the stairs in both directions—first thing in the morning and again at lunchtime. This plan wouldn't replace a balanced exercise program, but it could increase the muscles he used and energy he expended daily as a natural part of his life.

The results were encouraging. Bob timed his stair-climbing and began to average eight minutes a day, five days a week. Simply by taking the stairs at work, he accumulated an average of forty minutes of exercise or nearly an hour of bodily exertion per week. Just for fun Bob and I estimated the calories he burned each week by taking the stairs and were encouraged to see 360! Over the course of ten weeks, this single activity could burn 3,600 calories, roughly the amount of energy that must be expended to lose one pound; by staying with this one lifestyle change, Bob had the potential to lose five pounds in one year. Take that five-pound loss and multiply it by just five years, and it's easy to see how even that small change could add up over time.

Better than that, though, was this reality: As Bob continued his stair regimen, he noticed his lower body felt stronger and he felt more energetic during his workday. Most important, he felt great about his accomplishment. By making the decision to be active, he was inspired to ride his bike on weekends and drink more water. He still doesn't do as much conditioning and flexibility exercise as I'd like, but Bob has come a long way—and his back and health are the better for it.

As much as I would love for everyone to embrace thirty minutes of cardiovascular exercise, fifteen minutes of strength training, and fifteen minutes of flexibility and relaxation on a daily basis, this just isn't going to happen without major cultural change. Our lives are crammed with work and other commitments, not to mention all the effort it takes just to get through one day. But with a little imagination and creativity, anyone can find ways to work back into daily life more bodily exertion, which is such a natural part of being human.

Also I've never met a person who didn't feel better after exercising, even after moderate exercise. Our bodies were designed more for exertion and use than for being sedentary. Even people who resist the very idea of physical effort have to admit they feel good when it's over. So any step toward movement is a step in the right direction and will yield rewards.

With that happy thought in mind, consider how you can increase the amount of bodily exertion in your daily life. Remember that the goal here is to make physical activity a natural and unavoidable part of your life, like brushing your teeth. Look at the flow of a typical day:

- Do you have stairs in your home or at work? Even a decision as innocuous as using the upstairs bathroom can make a big difference.
- Where do you park when you go to the grocery store? Do you spend valuable time waiting for the perfect parking spot to open

39

up? Try parking as far away as is safely possible and walking a greater distance every time you shop.

- Do you have a friend or colleague you meet for coffee or lunch regularly? Suggest taking a leisurely walk together in a park or inside a mall to expend energy while you talk. In fact, inject walking into your life as much as possible, because walking is one of the most natural forms of exercise. Unless you're physically handicapped, your legs can propel you through every facet of your life.

Several summers ago, my mother lost ten pounds without really trying. She and my dad had visited Europe for the first time; over the course of a month, they walked practically everywhere they went to explore different towns and villages. Without making any adjustments to her diet—in fact, she probably ate a little more than usual—Mom came back to the States with looser-fitting clothes.

I had an eye-opening experience myself several years ago, when I walked day-in, day-out for one week on a vacation. My sisters and I had gone to a Huber family reunion in Montana, after which we walked and hiked through Glacier National Park. This was all done at a leisurely pace with no fitness goal in mind; when I returned to Nashville, my jeans had more breathing room. I'd lost weight and toned up muscles without even trying! I was especially amazed because at the time I'd been teaching group exercise in addition to running on a strict schedule. Looking back I see how I was naturally active throughout those days in Glacier Park—even more than as a fitness professional at home.

Another easy way to increase physical movement and exertion is to get away from the television. This one trapping of modern life has probably done more damage to our bodies and minds than any other product of the technological age. Unless a person is on a piece of exercise equipment, time spent in front of the TV is sedentary living at its worst. Seriously reducing TV time—or even better, getting rid of it all together—is a sure way to increase more active pursuits.

Before you think television deprivation is a huge effort, I must say that when I first experimented with TV-less living, I was amazed at how much better I felt and how much more time I had to do the other things I really wanted.

I recommend you try this: Make an agreement with yourself or your family that you'll live TV-free for one week. Then take a notepad and write down all the hobbies, outings, and areas of interest you'd like to explore if you only had the time. Highlight the ones that get you up and moving—better yet, things that get you out of the house. My list includes taking my dogs to obedience training, exploring antique shops, and browsing wonderful bookstores. Your list might include starting a vegetable garden, playing with the family, or getting together with friends you really care about but never see.

Now take that TV time and cash in on some of those life experiences. Enjoy a leisurely walk around the neighborhood. Ice-skate with your kids. Buy a basketball and shoot hoops at your local playground. Explore an interesting museum. Meander through an old junk store, browse the bookshelves of your public library. I guarantee this time will become cherished and golden. Once the TV withdrawal eases, you'll never want to go back to that wasted, sedentary life again.

These lifestyle adjustments might sound too subtle to make a difference in your health, especially if you're looking for changes in the weight and shape of your body. But remember Bob's experience of how small shifts add up over time? Keep reminding yourself that all the small steps move you toward wellness. The beauty of small adjustments is they're easy to do and tend to become a natural part of living. One day you'll realize that, almost without thinking about it, you've integrated more activity into your life.

That was the beauty of my grandparents' time. My grandpa wasn't trying to elevate his heart rate when he worked in the fields; his heart benefited naturally from what he did as a way of life. My grandmother wasn't trying to increase her bone density and muscle mass by doing loads of laundry through the hand-wringer washer or by carrying baskets of damp, heavy laundry to hang on the clothesline. Still, her body benefited from her labors.

Today's convenient privileges and comfortable luxuries don't mean much to people who don't have the strength and energy to enjoy them.

41

Now's the time to start using that small notebook mentioned at the end of the chapter on motivation. This is your daily wellness journal, a record of the changes you'll make in your life. As I said earlier, this log can be as simple or involved as you want. You can even record this in your Daytimer. Begin by daily noting the date, and under a category called ACTIVITY briefly describe how you were active that day. This valuable tool will help you stay accountable to a regimen all your own and give credit where credit is due.

I've kept my own records this way for a long time, and one of the greatest benefits is how it helps me stay focused. Next to ACTIVITY I'll write things like "hiked with client thirty minutes" or "did short run outside" or "walked on treadmill twenty minutes" and "walked JoJo" (my beloved Akita). Seeing in black and white what I do—or don't—keeps me mindful and motivated. In fact, such an account is just as valid and important as the checkbook used to keep track of spending or car maintenance record for assessing auto performance.

With this tool in hand are you ready to take a look at how you exercise? Remember, exercise is only one component of wellness. It's important, but no more so than any other subject in this book. So if you're at the same place my clients are when they pick up the phone to call me for an exercise plan, forge ahead. But if you're starting from scratch, increasing the activity in your daily life might be all you want to take on at this point. If that's the case, feel free to skip ahead to the next chapters while you get this first step toward regular exercise under your belt.

Whatever your situation, I'd rather encourage you to have success with a reasonable goal—even a small one, than to take on too much too soon (a very natural human tendency), get frustrated, and lack follow-through. Remind yourself: I'm just getting started, and I'm going to work from the inside out.

<hr />

Let us then, be up and doing with a heart for any fate; still achieving, still pursuing, learn to labor and to wait.
HENRY WADSWORTH LONGFELLOW IN "A PSALM OF LIFE"

How do we start? My initial sessions with clients ready for an exercise plan (and here's an understatement) are usually more subtle than expected. For example, we'll explore the different components of a well-rounded regimen and focus on some pretty subtle physical abilities like standing on one leg while isolating movement in the other. Or we'll learn to change the position of the pelvis by contracting the muscles of the torso.

Many clients first are surprised, relieved, or disappointed that our hour together won't leave them in a pool of gelatinous sweat. Then they wonder: Why focus on such seemingly small details?

That's a normal reaction, given the Olympian feats of fitness that so often represent exercise in our culture. But we'll not waste time on things that aren't important. As my clients learn, there's a great reason behind these methods. There's value in working from the inside of the body to the outside and, in the process, to developing strength and knowledge that can be used for a lifetime.

So start with that leap of faith to reach fitness goals from a different angle. It's an enjoyable process and delivers good results. If you begin to think you should be working out in more grandiose ways, think of what you're doing as building a house or buying a car. . . .

Imagine you have a nice piece of property for building that dream house—and the funds to do it. You would work with an architect to design what you want, say something functional and pleasing to the eye. Then you would hire a contractor or builder to bring the architect's design to fruition. Let's say the builder lays the foundation of the house and you check it out, as any concerned homeowner would. You look at the concrete and notice there are gaps or cracks. You study the foundation walls and notice they're not squared properly.

The builder listens to your concerns and says, "Well, there are a few problems here and there, but we can accommodate those imperfections as we go along."

Would you consider this to be an option, even for one minute? Of course not. You would say, "Every piece of this house relies on the soundness of the foundation, and it has to be made right before we add anything else to the structure."

43

Now imagine car shopping. You find a good deal on a car you like and take it to a trusted mechanic. The mechanic looks it over and says, "The engine is in great shape, the interior is beautiful, the paint job is perfect, but the frame is bent and the alignment out of whack."

Would you go ahead and buy this car without addressing the alignment issues? No, you probably would move on to a different vehicle, because bad alignment means tire problems, brake issues, and big repair bills in your future.

Foundation and alignment are terms that apply to the soundness of our bodies, just as they do to houses and cars. If anything, these terms take on much greater importance where our bodies are concerned, because our foundations can't be repoured or our parts replaced without a lot of pain, expense, and suffering. Therefore, foundational integrity and proper alignment of the body are essential ingredients to any exercise program; they affect the safety and effectiveness of both strength training and cardiovascular exercise, not to mention the huge impact on what we do with our bodies day-in and day-out when we aren't exercising.

For this reason it's important to address the way you stand and sit. These are the basics of your alignment, and just that—basics. You'll learn to be aware of, and possibly correct, the most common alignment problems that affect even the average person's posture. However, I can't recommend highly enough that you work one-on-one with a professional who addresses your specific postural analysis and stability training too.

I praise you because I am fearfully and wonderfully made . . .
PSALM 139:14

In order to assess your alignment you must know the three things that affect it most: the inherent symmetry of the human musculoskeletal system, your genetic tendencies, and your postural habits, which include the cumulative effect of any self-care or neglect, injury, or illness that you've sustained.

Your goal will be to move toward the body's inherent symmetry, within your inherited limitations, and reverse or at least improve the postural shortcomings most of us share. The amazing part of this process is that most people can start seeing very positive changes in appearance and body comfort by just becoming aware of basic posture cues.

Think of the human skeleton and how the bones line up. When God created Adam on the sixth day, he wasn't fooling around! Every bone, every joint, every joint function, and range of motion have purpose and perfection. Human beings truly have been designed from Creation to participate in and enjoy the abundance of life. From the twenty-six bones that make up the foot, to the top of the skull, there's symmetry and flow in the skeleton.

Misalignments happen when muscles pull the skeleton out of its perfect order, and this results when muscles become weak from disuse, shortened or atrophied by lifestyle, or tensed and imbalanced by a traumatic injury. Then there's a ripple effect throughout the body; other muscles tighten, shorten, or weaken as the body tries to compensate. Repetitive motions and weight-bearing exercise can add even more stress to any misalignment. The danger, then, of plunging into exercise without first looking for proper alignment is the same as for a house or car: The structure or mechanics will give in to their weakest link.

—∞∞∞—

We learn to do something by doing it. There is no other way.
JOHN HOLT, EDUCATOR

Now that you understand the importance of your alignment, imagine I'm your personal trainer. My first encouragement to you would be to work barefoot and in clothing that allows you to see the line of your body: ankles, knees, hips, lower and upper back, shoulders, neck, and head. Next, set aside thirty minutes for yourself, undistracted. You'll need to work in front of a full-length mirror, and you'll want to have a second, hand-held mirror at hand too. As you stand facing the full-length mirror, be kind to yourself. This is not an exercise in finding flaws. It's a step toward improving the way your body looks and functions.

First observe your legs and feet. For the purpose of standing in good alignment, your feet should be directly in line vertically with your hips or about five inches apart horizontally. Look from above and also in the mirror at the direction and position of your feet. Is one foot farther forward than the other? Be sure to place them evenly; notice if your feet tend to turn out or in. Ideally, the lines running from inside the feet (heel to big toe) should be close to parallel, with the toes slightly farther apart than the heels.

Now look at your ankles. Do they roll out or cave in toward each other? If they cave in, roll the arches of the feet away from each other, gripping the floor with the outside of the feet and pressing evenly through heels and toes. If your ankles tend to roll out, you'll need to grip the floor from the insides of your feet. Your goal is to have the ankle joint centered over the width of the heel.

Now check your hip-to-knee-to-foot line. Bend the knees slightly. Do the knees track over the feet and still line up with the hips? You want these body parts to flow in the same direction. Notice if the knees cave in toward each other as they bend, or if they splay. Bend and straighten several times slowly as you make the small adjustments necessary to maintain your hip-to-knee-to-foot line comfortably.

The changes you make probably won't feel natural at first, but they shouldn't hurt either. Remember, part of this exercise is to create awareness so your alignment improves.

Focus a little longer on the knees. Straighten them completely, noticing what it feels like to have them locked. Now soften those joints by bending or flexing the knees very slightly. This is a good, strong position for the knees to be in when standing, because when the knees lock, it causes tension in that area and usually puts a strain on the lower back. By flexing the knees slightly you can relieve that stress and engage the front of the thigh muscles (the quadriceps) for stability.

Turn sideways now to view your alignment from a different angle. Take a moment to reestablish your feet, ankles, and knees; then look for the natural curve in the lower back called the lordotic curve. This is the area often called "the small of the back," the part that curves inward. There's another curve in the upper back, called the kyphotic curve, between the shoulders; it curves or rounds outward. The spine curves once again in a second lordosis where the back turns into the neck, which of course supports the head. The goal is to maintain these natural curves while lining the skeleton up with the flow of gravity.

Adjust these three parts of the spine, starting with the lower back. Take one hand and find the base of your spine, the tailbone. With the other hand, locate the middle front edge of your pelvis, the pubic bone. Press against the tailbone, and squeeze your abdominal muscles, tilting the pubic bone forward and up. This action will flatten and possibly round the small of your back. Now reverse the action by pressing against your pubic bone. This will tilt the pelvis so that the hips stick out behind you and the lordotic curve of your back will increase. When tucking the pubic bone forward and up, you're engaging your abdominal muscles. When tilting the tailbone back and out, your back extensor muscles come into play.

Slowly change position back and forth, pressing against the tailbone and then the pubic bone to get a feel for the tilting action of the pelvis. Now cross your arms over your chest, getting them out of the way. Tilt your pubic bone slightly forward and up to find a neutral position for the lower back. Do not lose your lordotic curve altogether, just think of softening that curve. The goal is to find the solid, comfortable place that honors the natural curve of the lower back and supports it by engaging the abdominals. You do not want to exaggerate or eliminate the lower back curve, but rather find a neutral position that protects it.

Now drop your arms to your sides and face the mirror once again. Take a moment to reset your feet, knees, hips, and pelvis. Focus your attention on the rib cage and above. Drop your head and shoulders forward to round the upper back, exaggerating the kyphotic curve, then return to normal. Do this slowly a few times to feel the movement of your spine, shoulders, and shoulder blades. Come back to normal position, and gently pull your shoulder blades toward each other, engaging the upper back muscles. Then press your shoulders down, away from the ears. These upper back muscles, the trapezius and rhomboids, which make these actions possible, are your new best friends.

By engaging these muscles, lowering your shoulders, and collecting your shoulder blades together, you're opening the chest and improving the way you look and feel. You're not trying to imitate a military posture here, but rather neutralizing the rounded shoulders and upper back that most of us suffer from. When you've found the right place for those shoulder blades to live, gently arrange your head to ride above it all—in glory!

Now you'll need that hand-held mirror. Hold it in one hand and turn sideways again to the full-length mirror. Take a moment to reset your posture from toe to head. Hold the small mirror in the hand farthest from the full-length mirror to see what you look like from the side, with your head facing the same direction as your body. Drop an imaginary plumb line from head to toe. Your heels, knees, hips, shoulders, and ears should be in a line that flows with gravity.

Face forward, dropping your hand with the mirror to your side. Your lines should flow in this direction as well—head centered, shoulders down and slightly back, chest lifted and open, hips even, knees under hips, feet under knees. Notice how balanced and natural you look. You may feel strange in this position, but by simply regularly making yourself aware of it, you can begin to gravitate toward this good posture.

Every exercise in this chapter will employ these principles of alignment, and every day-to-day task will feel different because you've taken the time and care to address the foundation of your body. By simply being aware of these body alignment cues, you'll feel and see improvements in your posture. Also, you'll use this basic alignment as a foundation for the stability and strength exercises that follow.

However, the most practical and important application of good alignment is in your daily living. Next time you think of it, notice how you're positioned:

- Is your weight distributed evenly on both feet, or are you leaning into one hip and one leg?
- Are your knees locked as you stand in line at the grocery store, or are they slightly flexed and in line with the feet and hips?

- When you sit in your car, are your shoulder blades drawn together and down, or are they pulled apart, shoulders drooping, head and neck craning forward?
- When you sit at a desk to work, writing or using the computer, are you flowing with gravity, or is gravity pushing down on a spine that is not lined up to function efficiently?

These daily activities are perfect opportunities for mentally reviewing posture cues. As these cues become more natural and automatic, you'll notice that being out of alignment feels wrong; after the initial growing pains of this process of change, you'll wonder how you functioned as you had formerly.

Now that the groundwork has been laid, you can progress to the next phase of this exercise program—stability training.

⟨≈≈⟩

The body is a sacred garment. It's your first and last garment;
it is what you enter life in and what you depart life with,
and it should be treated with honor.
MARTHA GRAHAM

Structural stability is the foundation on which every physical task you perform rests. Stability training will not deliver body parts of steel or weight loss. It's about developing inner strength, strength that emanates from the core of the body. This phase of the training process will give you a solid place from which to work and ensure the safety and effectiveness of whatever additional physical efforts you make.

To a certain degree you depend on your stability all day long. When you walk, run, or climb stairs, you briefly rely on the ability of one leg to support your body weight. When you sit down and stand up, you depend on the stabilizing forces of your hip and knee extensors to move you around without falling over. And whether you sit, stand, or walk, your abdominal and back muscles constantly work to keep your torso upright against the pull of gravity.

Any time you increase your weight-bearing and athletic activities, you put added stress on your stabilizing muscles. These muscles—which control and support your ankle, knee, hip, torso, shoulder, and neck movements—are located below the superficial musculature on the surface of your body. The hip and shoulder rotator muscles are just two types of stabilizing muscles you can't see but depend upon. That's why it's a great mistake, and a common one, to jump into strength training and impact aerobics without first addressing these smaller, less obvious muscles. In fact, there's a big, although often unheralded pay-off in devoting time and attention to the muscles used in stability training: improved balance, the ability to isolate and control body movements, a sense of well-being, and safety (since nothing cuts off the well-intentioned exercise program faster than an injury).

Before beginning the exercises themselves, keep these things in mind too: The degree to which you need to work on stability depends a good deal on your fitness goals. Since I believe the most important goal is to be foundationally strong (so you can function easily and free of pain), I recommend exercises like the ones that follow. These can help you develop basic stability for any walking, hiking, or moderate running program. But if your personal fitness goals are sports-specific—like running marathons, body building, or competing in tennis, basketball, or other team sports, you'll need to focus more on the rotator cuff, torso, and hip and leg muscles. I'd also encourage you to seek one-on-one assistance with a qualified personal trainer. And I'd urge you to make an appointment for a thorough physical exam with your general practitioner. Run any exercise regimen by your doctor before you start, and if you feel any pain that surpasses normal muscle soreness from these exercises, discontinue the activity and seek professional assistance.

Now about these basics: I wish everyone would learn these ten exercises in elementary school and do them for the rest of their lives, because so much physical pain and suffering could be prevented. While injury is always a possibility with any movement, these exercises are so controlled the risks are minimal. Another benefit: You won't need any official equipment—just a stair step or ledge of some sort for three of the leg exercises, and, optionally, a full-length mirror as a great tool for checking alignment.

It's best to work the floor exercises on a well-padded, carpeted surface to protect your hands and knees. Also, wear a solid, laced shoe, such as a good walking shoe with some rubber tread on it, to support your feet.

Exercise 1—Pelvic Tilt & Reverse Pelvic Tilt

Since stability begins at the core of the body, in the muscles that move and support the spine, the most important point of this exercise is learning how to control and isolate pelvis and rib cage movement. It's great for mobilizing the back and is a building block for more advanced exercises like crunches and back extensions too. So think of this exercise as a warm-up and focus on the abdominal and back muscles.

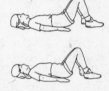

- Lie on your back with knees bent, feet flat on floor, hips width or so apart. Let your arms relax at the sides.
- Do a pelvic tilt by contracting your abdominal muscles to tuck your pelvis under, rolling the lower back into the floor, and tilting your pubic bone toward your rib cage.
- Do a reverse pelvic tilt by contracting your back extensor muscles to roll your lower back slightly off the floor. Done properly, this creates a hollow place, like a tunnel, between your lower back and the floor.
- Carefully repeat these 2 movements 15 times, feeling the position of the pelvis and spine change from a pelvic tilt to a reverse pelvic tilt.

Exercise 2—Abdominal Crunches

Contrary to popular belief, this exercise will not flatten your stomach or make your body a rippled vision of perfection. It will, however, strengthen one of your most important torso stabilizers—the abdo-minis rectus muscle.

It helps to fix an image in your mind of where this muscle is attached on the abdomen: from the lowest end of the pelvis to the middle of your rib cage. If you focus on the action of that muscle as a primary mover (torso flexion), you'll save a lot of time and achieve the great-est benefit. When a muscle contracts in the shortening phase of a joint action, the two points where it attaches get closer together. You've already experienced this with the pelvic tilt. By contracting the abdom-inal muscles, the pelvis tilts under—toward you—and gets closer to the rib cage. The crunch takes this shortening action one step further by moving the rib cage closer to the pelvis. The main thing, then, is to set the pelvis before you start crunching, and to avoid moving any-thing except the rib cage.

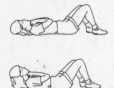

- Lie on your back with knees bent and feet on floor.
- Pelvic tilt to roll the lower back into the floor. This part of your body should not move again until you are done with this set.
- Make fists and place hands under your chin with elbows bent, arms resting on chest. This prevents pulling your head forward, and gets your arms out of the way.
- Contract your abdominals to move the ribs closer to the pelvis, rolling the head and upper back away from the floor and squeezing the muscle as if you are wringing out a washcloth.
- Lower your upper body toward the floor without relaxing tension on the ab muscles. Stop just short of contact with floor, then begin next repetition. (Breathe out as you curl forward on the exertion, breathe in as you lower back toward the floor.)
- Do this 10 to 20 times continuously. Do 3 sets, alternating this exercise with the Back Extensions.

Don't worry if your neck dictates how many crunches you can do; this is a common occurrence. Remember, your neck muscles are stabilizing the weight of your head against gravity when you do a crunch, which is a considerable feat. As you get stronger, both in the neck and abs, you'll be able to do more crunches—stronger neck muscles are a nice by-product of this exercise. Just remember what the primary focus of the crunch is: stronger abs with no extraneous movements, especially with the neck and head.

Exercise 3—Back Extensions

Have you ever heard that strong abdominals are good for your back? Well they are, but even more important are strong back muscles! The back extensor muscles (or erector spinae group) run like little cables along each side of the spine from the sacrum to the base of the head. To strengthen these muscles, this exercise has you performing the exact opposite action from the abdominal crunch—a spinal extension. One helpful hint: You might want a towel to put under your face for this exercise—depending on when you vacuumed last!

- Lie facedown on floor, legs extended and arms by your side. Rest the tip of your nose lightly on the floor, keeping your neck in a neutral position.
- Contract your back muscles to gently lift your upper body slightly away from the floor, then lower toward the floor and lift again. It's important that you avoid lifting too high, letting your feet come off the floor, or pulling back your head. Stay focused on a neutral neck position and imagine those cable-like extensor muscles working like pulleys to lift and lower your upper chest and shoulders.
- Focus on breathing out as you lift up and breathing in as you lower down.
- Do 10 to 15 repetitions, 3 sets, alternating with sets of crunches.

Exercise 4—Cross Lift on All Fours

Of all the exercises in this chapter, this is perhaps the best example of a simple one that can prevent or relieve pain. Because it works the back,

53

hips, and shoulders for balance and stability, it's a wonderful tool for general wellness too.

Be sure to wear something easy to move in when you do this one, work on a padded carpet or mat to cushion your knees, and work in front of a full-length mirror if you have one.

- Get on all fours (or your hands and knees) and place your hands directly under your shoulders and knees under your hips. Take a moment to set your back in a neutral position, shoulder blades set slightly together, lower back neither rounded nor sagging. Think of having your back even enough to balance a tray of iced tea.

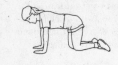

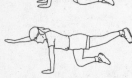

- Lift your right arm and left leg simultaneously to bring each limb to shoulder and hip level respectively. Hold for 2 full counts.
- Now repeat this with your left arm and right leg. Keep the limbs straight as you lift, without straining or pulling your back out of position. Think of floating the arm and leg up effortlessly. Do this entire sequence 10 times.

Exercise 5—Modified One-Legged Squat

For practicing the correct tracking of the knee over the foot, this exercise is fabulous. It also strengthens the quadriceps (muscles of the front upper leg) and buttocks.

You'll need a sturdy step that won't tip, or a stair or ledge to stand on for this and the next two exercises. You'll also need something to hold onto, which makes a doorway with a step or a staircase with a railing the perfect setting. If you feel any pain in the knee area, discontinue it until you can get some hands-on guidance. Otherwise . . .

- Stand sideways on the step, with your standing foot fully on the step but close to the edge, other foot even with the standing foot but totally free of the step or any other surface.

- Keeping the pelvis-hip line neutral and even, bend the standing knee just enough to lower the free leg toward the floor about three inches. Now straighten that knee to return to starting position. It's very important to watch the direction of the standing knee as it bends and straightens. Make sure it's tracking the direction of the foot, not caving in or bowing out. Also restrict any movement other than knee flexion. The pelvis should not rock and the torso should remain aligned.

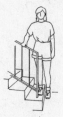

- Repeat this bending and straightening action 10 times, then change legs and complete the same number of repetitions. Do two or three sets, alternating legs accordingly.

Exercise 6—Outer Hip Strengthener

This exercise strengthens the main hip abductor (or gluteus medius) muscle, which worked as a stabilizer on the last exercise—only here that muscle is used as a primary mover.

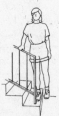

- Stand sideways on the step as before, knees straight, hips even, one leg fully supported by the step, the other completely free of it.
- Keep both legs straight (though not locked) throughout these movements, working from the standing hip alone. Without changing knee, foot, or torso position, hitch the free leg up a few inches by contracting the outer hip muscle of the standing leg. The only body part that changes position is the pelvis, as it lifts and lowers the free leg.
- Now reverse this, lowering the free leg three

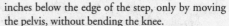

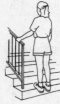

inches below the edge of the step, only by moving the pelvis, without bending the knee.

• Repeat this lifting and lowering movement up to 20 times; then reverse position (so the other leg becomes the standing leg) and repeat the entire sequence.

Exercise 7—Heel Raises

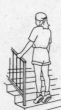

This is the last exercise to do on a step or ledge; it's a basic and familiar exercise for the back of the lower leg or calf muscles. The key is to think of the calf muscles being engaged in both the lifting and lowering stages of this exercise.

• Stand facing forward on the step with both feet hips' width apart and balanced on the edge of the step on the balls of your feet, with your heels extending off the step.
• Contract your calf muscles to push up as high as you can onto the balls of your feet on tiptoe, then reverse direction with control, lowering heels slightly below the level of the step.

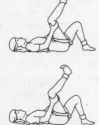

• Lift and lower in this manner, without pausing or hanging on the lowering phase, but rather working continuously 15 times.
• Do 3 sets of this exercise with brief rest periods (of 30 to 60 seconds) between sets.

Exercise 8—Ankle Point-Flex-Circle

This exercise is wonderful for developing strength and mobility of the ankle and lower leg. It appears to be a lot more subtle than it feels, so take your time building up to added repetitions.

• Lie on the floor on your back with both knees bent and feet flat on the floor. Lift the right leg toward your body, keeping the knee comfortably bent and supporting the leg with your arms.

- Point and flex your foot back and forth, working through as much range of motion as you can without moving the knee. Do this 10 to 20 times.
- Without resting, now circle your foot 10 to 20 times first one direction, then the other. Make the best complete circle you can each time.
- Lower this leg and foot carefully to the floor and repeat this entire sequence on the other leg.
- Since this exercise can be pretty intense, start by doing one or two sets of 10 repetitions on each action (point, flex, and circling) and build up to three sets of 20 (of each action) gradually.

Exercise 9—The Push-Up

The push-up has long been a basic of the strength-training repertoire, and there are many ways to do it: standing at a wall or against a countertop, from the knees, and of course, the full push-up done from the hands and feet.

The beautiful thing about the push-up is that it's a complete exercise, working to strengthen several muscles at the same time: The chest muscles (pecs) contract to bring the upper arm from a horizontal to vertical position against the resistance of your body. The muscles at the back of the upper arm (triceps) contract to control the bending and straightening of the elbows against the resistance of your body weight. The front shoulder muscle (anterior deltoid) assists the pecs in their work, and the abdominals work like crazy to keep the back from caving in to gravity. I could go on and on about the benefits of this one exercise, but I hope this is enough to convince you not to skip push-ups. (I had until I felt a certain responsibility as a fitness instructor to be able to do at least 10 push-ups from my knees.)

Today I complete 30 full push-ups every two days, and I love the fact that I can actually do this—as well as the results I get from it. The same can be true for you, even if you never felt very strong in your upper body. As with many of the things recommended in this book: If I can do it, anyone can. I know what it feels like to nearly fall on my face while trying to do a push-up from the knees. But I can promise that if you work on push-ups faithfully, you'll get stronger.

The principles for all types of push-ups are the same, but two versions are focused on here: the push-up from the knees and a modified standing push-up. Since many people aren't in correct alignment before starting, take your time getting into the correct position.

Push-Ups from the Knees

- On your hands and knees on the floor, place your hands several inches wider than your shoulders without moving them farther forward of your body.
- Now—and this is crucial for good form!—without changing your upper body position, walk your knees back and rest your body weight on the part of the thigh that's just above the kneecap. This takes the pressure off the kneecaps and arranges your body in a diagonal line from ear to shoulder, to hip, to knee.

- Bend your elbows out to the side and lower your chest directly between your hands, toward the floor. Stop when your shoulders are even with the elbows. Contract your chest and arm muscles to push up to starting position.

- Reset your hand position and knee position as needed to achieve the symmetry and angles shown in the exercise diagrams.
- Do 8 to 10 repetitions, and 2 or 3 sets, with rest in between.

Push-Ups Standing at a Wall

If you've ever had difficulty with push-ups from the knees, try this modified push-up at the wall in a standing position. I've had several clients eventually go from this modified push-up to the traditional sort, so don't think of it as a cop-out. It's really a building block.

- Stand in front of a wall with your arms lifted to just below shoulder level, elbows straight and palms flat against the wall. Slide the hands out wider by several inches and step your feet back a few inches so you're leaning into your arms against the wall.

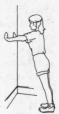

- Keeping your head and neck neutral, bend the elbows out to your side to lower your chest toward the wall, until your shoulders and elbows line up. Then push back to a starting position, fully straightening your arms.
- Do 8 to 10 repetitions and 2 or 3 sets.

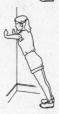

Keep in mind: The key to successful push-ups is maintaining certain angles. So when the elbows are bent, ready to push up, they should be in line with the wrists, over the hands. When lowering the body, the safest place to stop is short of going below the line of the elbows, which puts a strain on the shoulder. Finally, the torso and hips should remain in a neutral line, with head, shoulders, back, hips, and legs intersecting one line.

Exercise 10—The Backwards Push-Up

This last exercise works the back side of the body from head to toe. If your wrists don't get too tired, and to use your time more efficiently, you could alternate sets of these with sets of traditional push-ups.

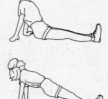

- Sit on the floor with your legs straight in front of you, hands on either side of your hips, palms down, fingers going out sideways.
- Slide your hands and arms straight back until your torso is leaning back, weight resting on your arms.
- Push into the floor with your hands and heels, lifting the rest of your body off the floor until you achieve a nice diagonal line from your head to your feet. Hold briefly and return to the floor.
- Do 5 to 8 repetitions, and 2 or 3 sets.

Once you've mastered the 10 exercises, this entire routine from start to finish takes about 20 minutes. Remember, the goal is to increase structural stability and function, and enhance your ability to be physically active. When done three times a week with rest days in between, and combined with regular physical activity (like walking for 20 to 30 minutes, 3 to 5 times a week), you could notice some changes in muscle firmness and density in 6 to 12 weeks.

Once you've devoted 12 weeks to this routine for stability, you can safely move ahead to a more advanced exercise regimen.

Cardiovascular Training: Exercise for the Heart

When Dr. Kenneth Cooper coined the word "aerobics" in the 1960s, the Fitness Revolution sprang into being. Suddenly the health benefits of walking, running, or biking—for periods of 20 minutes and longer at 60 percent to 80 percent of one's maximum heart rate—became newsworthy. Before long anyone could find all kinds of information about cardiovascular exercise and an endless stream of equipment and aerobic routines.

Now after 40 years or so, exercise has become a state-of-the-art science, and this fine-tuning for optimal fitness shows no signs of slowing down—nor should it. The Fitness Revolution has taught us much and will continue to reveal important information. But even the most capable exercise participants wonder if they're doing the right thing, when every few weeks there's a new study regarding the positive effects of a particular exercise regimen, done in a particular way, for a particular amount of time.

Woven underneath the myriad of prescriptions for aerobic training, strength training, and flexibility are basic, realistic fitness goals that apply to people of all ages.

So let's cut to the heart of the matter. Aerobic or cardiovascular exercise is good for the lungs, heart, and the entire cardiovascular system. By

60

engaging in regular aerobic exercise, a person will enjoy life-enhancing, and in some cases life-extending, benefits. These benefits include weight control, a decreased risk of heart disease and strokes, a decreased risk of developing certain forms of cancer, and protection from chronic conditions like diabetes and hypertension. After 40 years of research on the effects of cardiovascular exercise, the consensus is that participating each week in 3 to 5 aerobic workouts, each 20 minutes or longer, will help the average person enjoy the health benefits of cardiovascular exercise.

If every adult in our country followed this prescription faithfully, the impact on mortality rates, health care costs, and pain and suffering would be extremely positive. However, less than 25 percent of Americans follow through; this number has remained virtually unchanged, even through the fitness craze of the last several decades.

In an effort to encourage some kind of physical exertion by the other 75 percent, and based on studies showing benefits related to less formal exercise routines, the Centers for Disease Control and Prevention and the American College of Sports Medicine issued new guidelines in 1995 for physical activity: "Every U.S. adult should accumulate 30 minutes or more of moderate-intensity physical activity on most, preferably all, days of the week." The good news: This is compatible with the concept discussed earlier of "bodily exertion as a way of life."

But let's say you're ready to make a health specific commitment to regular aerobic exercise. Maybe you want to increase your cardiovascular benefits, improve your fitness level, lose weight, or any combination of these things. What's the next best step to take toward that goal?

First, keep in mind your unique abilities and capacities that cannot be compared to anyone else's. Then stay realistic. The most important thing is to find a method (or combination of methods) of continuous activity that you enjoy, and do that activity 3 to 5 times a week for 20 minutes or longer. Walking, running, swimming, bike-riding, stair-stepping, and aerobic dance are all examples of cardiovascular exercise.

Also keep in mind that you'll need a minimum of 5 minutes on both ends of your workout to warm up and warm down. So a 20-minute session takes about 30 minutes from beginning to end, and a 30-minute session takes a time commitment of about 40 minutes.

Commit to the amount of time you can do consistently, whatever works for your body and your schedule.

A common mistake people make in starting an aerobic training program is trying to do too much too quickly. They've been brainwashed to assume that more is always better. Well, more can be better, up to a certain point, but more becomes a moot point pretty quickly if the follow-through doesn't meet expectations. If you're just beginning a regimen, then, be willing to start small and add to it incrementally. There's nothing sadder for me than to watch someone give up on a program because they felt like a failure after setting the stakes too high. And keep in mind: Even though 5 weekly sessions, each lasting 45 minutes, sound better, 3 weekly sessions of 20 minutes each is nothing to sneeze at.

Even at a more goal-specific level of exercise, remember that everything you do adds up to your benefit.

<hr>

I used to think, the more the better, you can't run a good thing into the ground. Now I know that you can. People who run more than 15 miles a week are running for something other than cardiovascular fitness.

Dr. Kenneth Cooper in a personal interview

Another way to gauge how much aerobic training is right for you is by paying attention to the way your body feels. If you're running 30 minutes five times a week, how do your legs feel? Are your knees hurting? What about your feet and ankles—are they sore? Aches and pains may indicate that you're doing too much of the same activity, or that you need better shoes, or that the surface you're running on is too hard. You might benefit from shorter runs or alternating runs with a non-impact activity like swimming.

Let's say you go to the gym after work 3 days a week and spend 45 minutes on the Stairmaster. Again, listen to your body. How does your lower back feel? Are your knees constantly creaking and complaining? It might be time to cut the duration of your workout a little, or get out of the gym completely and enjoy a hike in the great outdoors.

Notice how other parts of your life are affected by the exercise routine you've chosen. Does your ability to fall asleep at night improve dramatically on the three days you go for a 20-minute walk? This could be a clue to increase your physical activity for most days of the week.

Maybe you take an aerobics class six days out of seven, at 90 minutes a pop. Are you exhausted when you wake up in the morning? Do your feet constantly hurt? Is your family life suffering at the cost of your workout routine? You may be overtraining.

It's very important to realize that, for all of its benefits, exercise does reach a point of diminishing returns. There are times when valid goals require more exercise, for instance when training for a race or athletic event, or accelerating necessary weight loss. But after 45 minutes of the same activity done at a moderate to high intensity, the chances of injury and overuse syndrome can surpass the benefits.

In fact, excessive exercise, regardless of the specific goal, is out of balance and carries its own risks. Life is too short to spend 2 hours a day on the treadmill. If you're motivated to accumulate long (meaning more than 45 minute) and frequent (more than five times a week) aerobic training sessions, be aware there's a trade-off. These long, tough workouts wear and tear the muscles and joints of the body. Dr. Kenneth Cooper points out: "Consistently excessive exercise is done for reasons other than health; it's been my experience that high-intensity, long-duration exercise has limited applications anyway. A person would have to have a very specific goal in mind to make this effort worthwhile."

Unfortunately, superhuman feats of fitness are what tend to get promoted in the media, especially as reflected in the lives of the rich and famous. In fact, celebrity worship and imitation is one of the most destructive influences in our culture. I wince every time I see a magazine article describing a famous personality's 2- or 3-hour daily workout regimen. That person might have a specific reason for such a regimen—stunts to perform in a movie, or just staying in that so-called "perfect" physical state for the limelight and the camera. But this isn't a measuring stick for real people. Celebrities pay a high price for maintaining the illusion of perfection.

You need regular exercise but regular rest too; you'll benefit most when time devoted to exercise is balanced with time for other pursuits with respect to the whole person.

My clients are frequently surprised when I tell them this idea—that health and fitness are not mutually inclusive terms. It's true that a measure of physical fitness is necessary for good health. However, it's possible to achieve a high level of physical fitness and still not be particularly healthy.

You can find examples of this in most any gym or workout center all over the country. The healthy-looking, lean and muscled body of someone who works out constantly is a reflection of many hours devoted to fitness training. Now this person may be quite physically fit. But does this person practice good nutrition, get adequate rest, and honor and balance the other elements necessary for overall health?

When determining the parameters of your own fitness routine, it's important to be honest with yourself about how it fits in with other components of a healthy lifestyle. Whether you choose to do 20 minutes of exercise 3 times a week, or longer sessions 5 times a week or more, some basic guidelines will help you maximize this investment of time and energy.

First, take at least five minutes to warm up by performing a slow and deliberate version of your intended activity. For example, if you walk or run for exercise, start with a slow, methodical pace, rolling through your entire foot as you put it down and increasing your speed gradually. Doing one set of the Heel Raises and/or Ankle Point-Flex-Circles from the Stability Exercises is an excellent way to warm up the legs for walking and running. If step aerobics or using the Stairmaster at the gym is your choice, add one set of the Outer Hip Strengthener to the others just mentioned. Again, start the activity at a slow pace and gradually increase your speed.

Try to spend the bulk of your session—after you warm up and until you cool down—in your target zone for beneficial exercise. To find this, you'll need to first estimate your resting heart rate by taking your pulse for one minute first thing in the morning upon waking naturally (without an alarm) and before you rise. Do this three different days and average the number. This is your resting heart rate. Now use this equation:

220 - your age = your maximum heart rate
Subtract your resting heart rate from your maximum heart rate.
Multiply that number by 0.6 (60 percent) and 0.8 (80 percent).
Add your resting heart rate back in to those two numbers.
The result will be the low and high boundaries of your target zone.

Probably the greatest challenge in finding your target zone is taking your pulse as you exercise. You have to be almost motionless to feel the pulse at your wrist or neck and then count, but stopping activity defeats the point of staying in the target zone.

I recommend trying, however, a couple of times during a typical workout to determine your baseline reference. Take the radial pulse at the wrist, rather than the carotid pulse at the neck, because it's safer to palpate. Use a stopwatch, count your pulse for 15 seconds, then multiply the number you get by 4. This estimates your heart rate per minute. Do this for 1 or 2 weeks to make sure you're in your target zone. After that, use your level of exertion as a point of reference.

Making a general reference for staying in the 60–80 percent target zone is known as "perceived exertion" and works on a scale from one to ten or from one to twenty. I prefer the one-to-ten method because it's so easy to picture. The question you ask yourself is, "How hard am I working on a scale of one to ten, with one being very, very easy and ten being very, very hard?" The range to aim for would be between four and six, which indicates you're, indeed, within your target zone.

Another way to gauge exertion is by whether or not you're breaking a sweat and how breathless you are. If, amid exercising, you can feel some moisture on your skin and talk enough to say a sentence or two, but not enough to carry on a full-fledged conversation, you're probably working at a good intensity.

By paying attention to your exertion level, you'll have a better chance of getting the biggest return for your investment of time and

65

energy. However, it's extremely important that this part of your program remain enjoyable. Some people have a greater desire to huff and puff and sweat than others. If you don't fit into that category, you may end up working at a level three or four of perceived exertion, and that's fine. The main thing is to keep your aerobic activity as something to look forward to, as it should be.

After your 20 minutes or longer in the target zone, take a good 5 to 10 minutes to cool down. This simply means backing off the intensity to let your heart rate drop gradually and let your body start to cool. Always rehydrate after you exercise to replace lost fluids. Then follow this part of your workout with a strength-training session or a few flexibility exercises as you continue to cool down.

Strength-Training

Someone once said trying to lose weight by restricting calories alone, without the help of regular exercise, is cruel and unusual punishment. I'd take this one step further and say trying to even maintain weight without the benefit of regular exercise, including strength training, is difficult indeed.

As beneficial as aerobic training is for weight control and health, I'd be hard-pressed to say it's more important than strength training.

Fortunately, you don't have to choose one over the other. Together they make a beautiful team, and even the busiest schedule can accommodate a handful of strength-conditioning exercises on a regular basis.

My personal experience with the extraordinary benefits of being physically strong has a lot to do with my enthusiasm. I know what it's done for me, and I've never worked with a client—especially a woman—who didn't blossom like a beautiful flower after exploring the potential for strength.

I didn't focus too much on strength work until I met the man I eventually married. I was an aerobics fiend at the time, teaching at least ten fitness classes a week, working with clients, and doing my own running program. John was an athletic trainer with years of weight-lifting experience but no particular zeal for cardiovascular workouts.

When we started dating, we also started working out together—and I got a serious dose of down-to-earth strength training right off the bat. Never having excelled at this, I expected the worst. Instead, I experienced one of the greatest discoveries of my life. Strength training made me feel wonderful. My body developed a balance and substance like never before, my energy and stamina increased, and my running got easier.

In the next year, I actually decreased my aerobic training by a third and, without adjusting my caloric intake at all, lost a few pounds. But the real thrill was feeling strong all over for the first time in my life. I'd been working out—one way or the other—for years. Suddenly, in my thirties, I was capable of things I couldn't do in my twenties. I went from barely being able to squeeze out 8 modified push-ups to doing 3 sets of 10 full push-ups several times a week. I'd never gotten close to pulling my body weight over a bar, but I gradually became capable of an unassisted pull-up from a dead hang. This was exciting stuff for someone who never felt particularly strong, especially through the upper body.

Most of the women I work with come from a similar background. They may have accomplished the laudable goal of exercising their hearts regularly, but for one reason or another dismissed strength training as not important or interesting.

Here's the great beauty of strength training and why it's too important to miss: Weight training combined with reasonable aerobic training gives you the best results for keeping in shape. It works like this: Every one of us begins to lose muscle mass as a natural part of the aging process starting in our twenties. As muscle mass decreases, metabolism also slows down and more body fat develops. This process happens quietly and sometimes escapes notice for years—maybe because the number on the scale might stay the same, even though changes are happening in body composition. This can happen because muscle mass weighs more, but takes up less space, than fat. Eventually, as muscle mass gradually decreases and stored fat increases, you see the weight gain—and it feels like it happened overnight.

Since your body uses 30 to 50 calories a day to sustain each pound of muscle on your frame, think of how you can bump up your metabolism with strength training! Others have in the medical community, fitness organizations, and the public at large—at least more so than in the past. The American College of Sports Medicine has added twice-weekly resistance (strength) training for all major muscle groups to their revised exercise recommendations in 1990. Also, old bodybuilding images, and the misunderstanding of what strength training accomplishes, are being positively rescripted. Women are less concerned about the myth of bulking up today than they were five years ago. They're also less apt to forego weight training because they're obsessed with aerobics, aerobics, aerobics to burn calories. This is a good trend.

⸻∞⸻

It's not what you do, it's how you do it.
TOM PURVIS

My career in wellness has been strongly influenced by another trainer and physical therapist who has revolutionized the field of strength training. His name is Tom Purvis, and he's known in fitness circles as the Kenneth Cooper of strength conditioning.

Tom is one of those rare individuals possessed with equal amounts of natural talent and the determination to improve on it. He's constantly challenging his own beliefs about training, and in doing so brings the art of training to a new level for everyone. His observations on old-school resistance training and innovative technique have put him in a class by himself.

Tom's philosophies about training and working the body from the inside out have been a foundation for my own approach with clients. I'd be remiss not to give him credit for that. His hands-on style of teaching how to perform muscle actions also gives me reason for not trying to teach strength training beyond the basic stability exercises we have already covered. The nuances of alignment and muscle isolation are too subtle and individually unique, especially when resistance is added in the form of weights. I do highly recommend working with a certified personal trainer or other fitness professional for guidance in strength training, and in the meantime using the following as a quick overview of the major muscle groups and benefits of strengthening them.

By doing the stability exercises from earlier in this chapter, you're already acquainted with many joint actions and muscle movements. Think of how every time you flex, extend, or rotate a body part, you're using your muscles—and how those muscles provide you with movements you take for granted. Now think of how your ability to engage in physical activity is completely dependent on the strength of those muscles to support your structure and move you around. Whether you lift babies, grocery bags, or dumbbells, the greatest benefit of physical conditioning is increased strength and mobility. With that in mind, look at the major muscles of the body and how they're used.

The Lower Leg Muscles

Every time you put your feet on the ground and walk, you rely on the muscles of the lower leg: the calf muscles (or gastrocnemius and soleus) in the back, and the shin muscle (or tibialis anterior) in the front. The calf muscles give you the ability to push your heels off the ground and come up on the balls of your feet, a motion you make with every step or whenever you stand on tiptoes. The shin muscle, considerably smaller and weaker than the calf muscles, flexes the foot toward the front of the body. You engage this muscle every time you lift your foot to tap it to the beat of good music.

Together, these muscle groups work in beautiful symmetry to propel, support, and balance you. So when you strengthen these lower leg muscles, you not only improve your athletic ability and mobility, but prevent injury. If walking, running, or aerobic dance are your activities of choice, you've a vested interest in maintaining the balance and strength of the calf and shin; the Heel Raises and Ankle Point-Flex-Circle exercises can help.

69

The Upper Leg and Hip Muscles

Body movement from the waist down is facilitated by the substantial thigh muscles of the upper leg working together with the largest muscles of the body, the gluteals or buttocks. The front of the thigh muscles (or quadriceps) straighten the knee and help flex the hip. (Think of the motion involved in kicking a ball.) The back of the thigh (hamstring) muscles provide the opposite function, bending the knee and extending the hip (now imagine standing on one foot and trying to touch your heel to your buttocks). The outer hip (or abductor) muscles provide movement away from the body, while the inner thigh (or adductor) muscles pull the leg towards the midline of your body.

These beautifully designed muscles work separately and in unison to help you walk, run, jump, and scoot side-to-side; by keeping the upper leg strong, you ensure your ability to stay active and injury-free. People who play team sports, tennis, or racquetball, or do any kind of regular impact aerobic training like running, benefit greatly from a well-balanced strength routine for these lower body muscles.

The best reason for keeping these muscles strong, however, is simply the ability to function. You know what I mean if you've ever watched an elderly person struggle to get up out of a chair. This picture is a perfect example of a functional need to maintain muscle tone and strength.

Several years ago I had the wonderful opportunity of working with a 91-year-old man. His main goal was to be able to get up from a seated position unassisted and walk well enough to play a few holes of golf. One of the exercises we did together was getting up from a seated position and sitting back down in a controlled manner to increase the strength of the buttocks and thighs. My client made significant strength and stability gains and was able to get back on the golf course to his (and everyone else's) delight.

Your Torso

Now what about the muscles that support the torso, the abdominal and back extensor muscles? These allow you to flex, extend, and rotate the spinal column, stabilizing the torso with every move you make:

when you bend down to pick something from the floor, when you turn to look behind you as you back the car out of the driveway, and even when you keep your torso erect as you stand and sit and move around.

One of the drawbacks to a sedentary lifestyle is that muscle mass of the upper body simply doesn't get enough use. Considering that, and the fact that almost everyone experiences a debilitating back episode at some point, this is the part of the body where strength training should begin. Fortunately, these muscles respond beautifully to even the simplest strength routine, like the Abdominal Crunches and Back Extensions.

The Upper Body Muscles

Now think of the large chest muscles (or pectorals), which fan across the ribs and cross your shoulder joints. The pectorals' primary action is to move upper arm toward the chest. These muscles allow you to wrap your arms around someone you love. They also make it possible to push against heavy objects, like a refrigerator you want moved or a stalled car you need to get out of traffic. If you've been doing push-ups, you know exactly where these muscles are and how good it feels to develop strength in this part of the body.

To balance any chest exercise, you must, must, must, strengthen the upper back. The muscles of the back look like a beautiful patchwork quilt with many overlapping layers. The trapezius starts at the base of the skull and forms a kite-like shape as it connects to the shoulders, shoulder blades, and mid- to upper-spine. This muscle elevates the shoulders (a shrugging motion), pushes them down, and moves the shoulder blades together.

Underneath the trapezius, running from the spine to the shoulder blades, are upper back muscles called rhomboids—and they help you pull your shoulders back and down, plus allow you good posture and back strength.

Learning how to strengthen these upper back muscles single-handedly saved my career as a musician. Years of curling my arms around the fiddle had resulted in trauma to my upper back. But the stress and

71

pain were completely reversed when I started a comprehensive upper-body strength training program. Although it's by no means a complete back routine, the Cross Lift on All Fours is a good exercise for this part of the body.

Now to the largest muscles of the back, your pulling and rowing muscles: the latissimus dorsi, or "lats." These magnificent muscles fan out around the sides of the torso from the base of the spine and attach to the front side of the upper arms. The wonderful V-shaped back of a swimmer shows an example of well-developed lats. However, most of us haven't fully maximized the strength of these muscles day-by-day. The easiest way to visualize the lats in action is to picture someone doing a pull-up, pulling the start-cord on a lawn mower, or yanking a stubborn weed out of the ground.

This may seem like an extreme case for developing functional strength, but I think the ability to pull up one's body weight is a reasonable conditioning goal. Who knows? Being able to pull yourself out of a ditch or off the edge of a cliff could save your life someday. But whether the ability to do a full pull-up is in your future or not, there are many ways to build strength and improve the function of these fine muscles, and you'll love the way your body feels when you've accomplished this too.

Your Shoulder and Arm Muscles

The last muscle group to mention here for the purpose of basic strength training are the muscles of the shoulders and arms. The anterior (front), medial (middle), and posterior (rear) deltoid muscles cover the shoulder joint like a shoulder pad. Together with the muscles of the rotator cuff, the deltoids enable shoulder movements that include lifting your arms to the front, side, back, and overhead, plus circling them all the way around. When you hold a baby or a bag of groceries in front of you at arm's length, you rely on the strength of these front shoulder muscles; when you use a backhand stroke in tennis, you're engaging the back muscle of the shoulder. Lifting both arms to shoulder level, directly out to the sides, is an example of the middle shoulder muscles in action.

Strong, healthy shoulder function is something you don't want to take for granted, whether you're hitting tennis balls, picking up children, or reaching overhead to put something on a shelf.

The large muscles of the upper arm are the biceps (in front) and triceps (in back). The biceps' primary function is to bend the elbow as when you pick up or pull things. The triceps' main function is to straighten the elbow as when you push things away, up, or down. When you pick up a bucket of water with one hand, bending the elbow and holding it steady, you use the biceps; when you straighten the elbow against resistance—throwing a softball, for example— you use the triceps. The results of strength training for these muscles, and those of the shoulder, can be seen and felt, in a short period of time.

The muscles of the forearms (lower arms) aren't considered part of the major muscle groups, but I always include forearm exercises as a part of the strength training process. For one reason, there's an increasing incidence of overuse and carpal tunnel syndrome, which indicates a need for more forearm strength, especially for people who work with computers or do highly repetitive movements in their jobs.

Mind Your Muscles

Now that you've waded through the major muscle groups and how they function, you might feel overwhelmed at the prospect of taking on a strength training routine. Let me assure you that after learning a few basic exercises, a comprehensive workout can take less than 30 minutes to complete, and two sessions a week are enough to develop musculature, with an additional session each week for significant gains.

Can you tell that strength training is one of my favorite things to go through with a client? It's because I know how it can put you in touch with your body, increasing not only body awareness, but self-esteem too. More than that, strength training can actually unlock the potential for being fit and strong in all areas of life, not just while exercising.

73

Flexibility

When I was young and foolish (or maybe I should say younger and more foolish) I wanted to achieve the flexibility of a ballerina. I can remember taking "Intense Stretch" classes at the Jane Fonda Workout Studio while visiting my parents in California, striving to attain the pretzel-like contortions of the instructor, who appeared so agile I sometimes wondered if she had any bones in her body.

Fortunately for my joints, I never achieved the ballerina standard demonstrated in athletic and fitness events. I have, however, settled into a state of functional flexibility—a healthy goal for most people. I say healthy, because the effortless body movements of a dancer, figure skater, or gymnast are beautiful to watch, but their level of flexibility is a perfect example of a very goal-specific endeavor. The standards of their sport demand, ultimately, a sacrifice of joint stability and physical wellness later in life. Ask professional dancers over the age of 40 about the price paid for such noodle-like, agile beauty: big-time joint pain and deterioration.

Flexibility for mere mortals simply means enjoying normal range of joint motion function. If you've ever had an opportunity to play with a model skeleton, you know what I mean. See how the joints of the body have certain boundaries of movement? For instance, the elbow and knee each are capable of bending until the lower part of the limb comes into contact with the upper part (so the forearm touches the biceps, and the calf touches the hamstrings). Yet neither joint goes the other direction beyond extending to a straight line. Or look at the shoulder and hip joints—each examples of ball and socket joints, which can flex, extend, abduct (move away from the body's axis), adduct (move toward the body's axis), and rotate. There's a degree of motion in these joints that's healthy and reasonable—and then there's a degree that's not healthy, that actually threatens the stability of the joint (for instance to allow for splits in all directions through the hip joints).

74

This degree of motion for the joints makes stretching for flexibility a standard component of exercise routines. While stretching can help you regain or maintain normal joint range of motion, this is another area of personal fitness that can benefit greatly from one-on-one professional guidance—because stretching can be taken to extremes.

From a purely functional standpoint, there are some standard joint movements that everyone is capable of—movements reasonable to attain and maintain. These are the flexibility exercises I recommend you do at the end of your workout, when your muscles are warm and pliable. Or do these exercises at least near the end of a day that includes physical activity. Work at your own pace within your personal boundaries; by no means should any of these exercises cause pain. Modify your position as you need to, or discontinue the exercise altogether if necessary.

Lower Leg and Hamstring Release

I rarely run into a client who has too much hamstring flexibility. In fact, usually there's a problem with tight hamstrings, accompanied by lower back pain, because of so much time spent sitting—at work, in the car, or in front of the television.

The problem is when you sit with your knees bent, your hamstrings are in a shortened position. Unless you counter that with exercise and movement, the hamstrings tend to atrophy and shorten over time and pull on the pelvis.

How do you know if your hamstrings are too tight? Sit on the floor with your legs straight in front of you with your torso upright, while maintaining a normal lower back curve. If you find this position difficult, the Hamstring Release will help you become more limber and develop strength and joint balance at the same time:

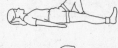
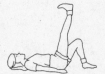

- Lie on the floor on your back with both knees bent, feet flat on the floor. Extend the right leg out on the floor, keeping the left knee bent and the left foot firmly planted.

75

- Straighten the right knee and flex the top of the foot back toward you as you carefully lift the leg off the floor. Press firmly into the floor with the left foot as you do this.
- Hold the right leg in the most upright position you can achieve without changing pelvis position, and without letting the knee bend or the foot relax.
- Keep pressing the left foot into the floor as you concentrate on lengthening the back of the right leg. Maintain this position for 30 to 60 seconds, or less if your leg tires.
- Repeat this entire sequence with the other leg.

Note: It's so easy to mistake a hamstring release for a lower back release, which is why I don't encourage pulling back on the lifted leg with the arms. You can, however, use your hands to support the leg, if you promise not to pull on it.

Quadriceps and Hip Flexor Release

The quadriceps and hip flexor muscles, like the hamstrings, also lose flexibility over periods of inactivity or being in a seated position too much of the time. The quadriceps work not only to extend the knee, but, along with the hip flexor, flex the hip. Sitting in a chair is an example of the hip being in a flexed position. There are many ways to release and lengthen these muscles, but it's important to avoid compressing the knee joint in the process—which is why this exercise works well:

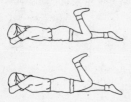

- Lie facedown on the floor, with your forehead resting on your hands. Bend one knee, pulling the heel toward the back of the upper leg.
- Contract your abdominal muscles to tilt your pubic bone into the floor. Then lift the knee slightly off the floor, without moving the pelvis.
- Hold for 10 seconds and lower to relax, keeping the knee bent. Do this 3 times for a total of at least 30 seconds, up to 1 minute.

Low Back Release

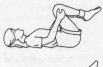

For back pain sufferers, or preventive medicine to maintain a healthy back, this is standard exercise fare:

- Lie on your back on the floor, with knees bent and feet flat on the floor. Draw one knee at a time toward your chest, supporting both legs by placing your hands under the knees.
- Contract your abdominals to roll your upper body forward, gently squeezing your body into a tight ball, and hold the position for 5 seconds. Be sure to move your upper body and lower body toward each other with your abdominals rather than by pulling with your arms.
- Release the upper body back to the floor, as you continue to hold your knees toward your chest. Repeat this 2 or 3 times for at least a full minute. Release your legs back to starting position one at a time when you are through.

Shoulder Release

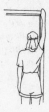

Many people tend to have an imbalance in the muscles that connect at the shoulder, and generally this is a combination of tight pecs and weak upper back muscles. But many daily activities only aggravate this imbalance: driving a car, working on a computer.

You can check your shoulder flexibility by lying flat on your back and raising your arms up and back behind you, to rest on the floor. Can you reach and maintain this position comfortably? The following exercise is one of my favorite shoulder openers.

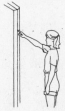

- Stand in front of a doorway with your right arm in front of you at shoulder level, fingertips

77

on the doorjamb. Walk your fingers up the doorjamb, keeping your arm straight.

- Walk the rest of your body forward as the arm reaches comfortably overhead until you are standing in the doorway with the arm straight and fully extended. Hold this position and breathe normally for at least 30 seconds and up to one minute. Release backward in similar fashion and repeat with other arm.

Remember, these flexibility exercises are like everything else covered so far: You'll get results based on the energy and concentration you put into each effort. Be willing to take small, consistent steps toward a greater purpose than mere appearance. Give yourself credit for whatever efforts toward physical activity you make. There will be times when it's easier to exercise than others, and it's natural to get off track for a while. But do get back. Try to think of exercise as just one of many investments you make in your life.

In fact, remind yourself that the most beneficial aspect of exercise is the connection it makes between body and mind. Every time you lace up your walking shoes, perform an exercise, or enjoy a stretch, you have an opportunity to dialogue with your body. It's a gift to be able to do all these things. Maintaining your body with mindful care and attention is an investment in your future well-being. It also benefits the people who love you. Everyone deserves to have time and energy to devote to this important part of being healthy.

The Power of Choice

Things you can do every day to impact your well-being

- **Keep in mind what's truly healthy and what's Fitness Revolution hype** as you contemplate what kind of exercise to include in your life and what results you want. Certainly, between the unrealistic body types, skimpy clothing, and vast array of machines and gadgets purporting to keep you fit, there are plenty of reasons to feel discouraged. But you can learn to observe these fitness industry images with a degree of detachment: Remind yourself daily that the best reason to exercise is to stay healthy, and that you already possess everything you need to be physically active as a way of life.

- **Keep track of your efforts in your daily wellness journal or Daytimer.** This record can help you fine-tune your approach to exercise by showing you what works best for your success and when. Which days of the week lend themselves to a 20-minute walk? What time of day best accommodates one set of floor exercises? The walks, runs, and exercises I've done and recorded in my daily wellness journal also show me the big picture—where I've been and where I'm going with my exercise program. Another benefit: It's not only affirming but motivating to give yourself credit for any positive effort you make toward better health.

- **Make deals with yourself**—another great tool for sticking with a program. On those days when you just don't have the desire to tackle a 20- to 30-minute walk, give yourself permission to do 5 minutes and let yourself off the hook. I can't count the number of

79

times I've gotten myself out the door on a 5-minute deal and ended up taking a 30-minute run. Getting started one day at a time is the most important step toward physical activity as a way of life.

- **Learn more about your incredible body.** I highly recommend *The Anatomy Coloring Book* by Wynn Kapit and Lawrence M. Elson as a resource for information and inspiration. Pick up a copy at the bookstore, treat yourself to a wonderful set of colored pencils, and have some fun while you develop a new level of respect for the vehicle that houses your heart, mind, and soul.

- **Without a huge investment of time and money, find a qualified fitness professional** to help design just for you a safe and effective exercise routine. Today, thanks to excellent certification programs and high industry standards for personal trainers, it's easier than ever. Many trainers will work a handful of sessions to help someone get started, then be available for follow-up as needed. When you're ready to take on a comprehensive regimen, look for someone with certification from ACSM (the American College of Sports Medicine), NASM (the National Academy of Sports Medicine), ACE (American Council on Exercise) or one of the other nationally recognized organizations that teach and certify fitness professionals.

- **Give some thought to making exercise enjoyable.** It's essential to have some measure of joyful anticipation for whatever activity you choose, otherwise it simply won't become a consistent part of your life. For me, running with my sister or one of my dogs is always more compelling than running alone; being outside and enjoying nature as I exercise is also important. What's important to you? What aspects bring you delight? Tap into those things.

Four

Food and Water

*It seems to me that our three basic
needs, for food and security and love,
are so entwined that we cannot think
of one without the other.*

MARY FRANCES KENNEDY FISHER FROM *THE ART OF EATING*

In the poignant and bleak 1983 film *Testament,* a brief scene depicts the full spectrum of our human need for food. This made-for-TV movie dramatizes the aftermath of a preemptive nuclear strike on the United States in a small community well outside of San Francisco. Jane Alexander plays the mother of three who holds her family together the best she can in the face of slow but sure death by radiation poisoning. Her husband, played by William Devane, travels on business to San Francisco on the fateful day, never to return.

Jane, her children, their neighbors, and friends struggle to survive a life that's suddenly turned into a nightmare, trying to bring normalcy to an existence that will never be normal again. A scene late in the movie shows Jane standing by the kitchen counter, eating the last few bites of peanut butter out of a jar. She's not slept in days. She wears a sweater that her husband wore the day before the nuclear strike—his scent on it is the last part of him left to her. She's buried her youngest and oldest children; she's exhausted and lonely, in a place beyond sadness, but for this moment she experiences a small measure of comfort.

Carefully, she scrapes the last bite of peanut butter from the jar. Thoughtfully, she raises it to her mouth on the end of a wooden spoon. She chews the peanut butter, feeling all of the texture and flavor on her tongue and in her mouth. For a brief moment her hellish reality retreats as she satisfies one of her human needs—hunger.

As human beings we share basic needs. From the day we're born and lifted to our mothers' breasts to the day we breathe a last breath, we have a relationship with one of those needs—food. The connection we have to the ritual of eating and satisfying hunger is more constant and long-lasting than many friendships. It's one of the most natural and pleasurable functions of our daily life. We eat alone or with others. We gather around a table to break bread, or celebrate birthdays, anniversaries, holidays, and commemorate death with food. Even our business functions revolve, frequently, around food.

Yet for all our common and universal involvement with eating, food, and the way each of us relates to it, is also very personal and unique. You develop individual likes and dislikes. You grow into patterns and habits very much your own. You learn what agrees with your stomach and what doesn't. You find, over time, what foods really make your mouth water. As with so many areas of life, your relationship with food becomes part of your personal history, a reflection of your personality and a blueprint for your health.

Ultimately, each person must make peace with food: The availability of it, the sensual pleasure it provides, and the miracle of how it nourishes every cell in the body are some of life's great blessings. Yet how often this is forgotten in our culture of fast-food restaurants and calorie-counting guides! What an irony that in a land of plenty, food has become a mixed blessing and the noneating of food (or dieting) has become a multibillion-dollar industry.

Think of what that means for a minute, this odd challenge of our times. From the beginning of time to the twentieth century, the growing, gathering, and preparing of food was the life work of most people. Even my grandparents relied on the grocery store for very little other than flour, sugar, and salt. My Grandma Huber canned and preserved everything that grew on the farm, never knowing what the next harvest would or wouldn't bring; sitting around the table to say grace before each meal was a daily ritual. This way of living and experiencing food was rooted in centuries-old human behavior and tradition.

Today's basic needs for nutrition and the blessing of good food haven't changed from my grandparents' time. But behavior and experience with food has, and not always for the better. Today people eat alone—and a lot: while standing over the kitchen sink, driving, sitting at a desk and working, or lying in front of the TV. When people do eat together, they eat faster, with less time for conversation, less etiquette, and generally less gratitude than in previous generations. People also buy more food that's refined and processed to the point it doesn't resemble food at all; indeed it's become less nutritious and more fattening. In fact, the fat-free and sugar-free foods bought to control weight often provide little nutrition and a bigger calorie punch than imagined.

The insidious increase of obesity and weight-related illnesses in our culture are a reflection of our modern lifestyles. For instance, the one meal you pick up at the drive-through window of a fast-food restaurant can equal an entire week's worth of fat calories. But the endless parade of diet plans, weight-loss pills, and expensive methods for trimming down haven't helped reverse this trend. If anything, the glut of diet products has swelled the tide of frustration and discontent. No wonder so many people today have lost the simple pleasure of eating.

Invariably, when I work with a new client, there are questions about food, diet, and weight control. How could there not be? For many years there's been an unfortunate tendency in our culture to infuse the subject of eating and weight control with magical thinking and mystery. But there's no substitute for plain old common sense. I can tell you from my own struggle, and from the numerous clients I've worked with on these issues, this area of our lives begs to be simplified.

My philosophy about eating is based on the sum of my personal and professional experience with food and on basic facts about nutrition. I encourage you to take whatever you can from my insights and factor in your own uniqueness. The way you handle this area of life has everything to do with how you feel, how much you weigh, and how healthy you are. My hope is you'll be able to make peace with food and return this essential part of living to the simple blessing God intended it to be.

The supple soul is one who joyously anticipates sitting down to the heavenly banquet—and who is able to do so with exuberant unconcern for whether or not the bread is buttered or the milk is 98 percent fat free.

MARY LOUISE BRINGLE FROM "CONFESSIONS OF A GLUTTON"

The cornerstone of a common-sense approach to food is compassion for one's self. By this I mean gentleness, forgiveness, patience, and self-love. Very few people haven't felt traumatized and ashamed over what they've eaten or not eaten. But society-driven, self-inflicted abuse must end before making a lasting improvement in the relationship with food. It's essential to experience real healing with food issues, and only each one of us can initiate the process.

It's important to acknowledge there will always be room for improvement in your eating habits. I've adjusted and tweaked my nutritional choices for many years and still want to do better in some areas. By treating myself with compassion, though, I remove that all-or-nothing thinking and those unrealistic expectations from my shoulders, and this is a much healthier mind-set. This means knowing that setbacks and interruptions to the best-laid diet plans are normal. So give yourself credit for even trying to improve this aspect of your lifestyle. So many people ignore it altogether or never try.

Also, consider dropping the term "dieting" from your vocabulary—permanently. Staggering evidence shows diets don't work, and most people who lose weight by dieting are doomed to gain it back. You can impose only so much structure in your daily life, so instead of dieting, think about lifestyle changes and healthier choices across the board. Then as you attempt to improve these choices, recognize how crucial it is to embrace the joy of eating.

You'll notice on this topic what minimal reference I make to calories and fat grams, and the endless caloric equations and percentages. Enough information on calories is readily available to those who seek it, written by experts in the field, and I find the equations can become mind numbing. I've also found that general parameters of healthy eating are easier to grasp. That's why I like the U.S. Department of Agriculture (USDA) Food Guide Pyramid (see page 93) and the chart (see page 87) suggesting specific guidelines based on age, gender, and activity level—and I'll refer to these resources frequently.

I'm convinced eating healthfully is a lot simpler than it's made out to be. Most of us can benefit greatly by simply understanding the following nutritional basics.

	Less Active Women, Older Adults	Children, Teen Girls, Active Women, Less Active Men	Teen Boys, Active Men
Calories	About 1,600	About 2,200	About 2,800
Grains	6 *	9 *	11 *
Vegetables	3	4	5
Fruits	2	3	4
Milk Group	2-3 **	2-3 **	2-3 **
Meats	2, for a total of 6 ounces	2, for a total of 6 ounces	2, for a total of 7 ounces

* Strive for at least three of these servings from whole grain foods
** Women who are pregnant or breast-feeding, teenagers, and young adults to age 24 need three servings

From *Eating Well, Living Well*, The Wheat Foods Council

∽∽∽

You cannot have your cake and eat [it] too.
MIGUEL DE CERVANTES SAAVEDRA IN *DON QUIXOTE*

Over the past thirty years the media has endlessly focused on Americans and their weight gains. Billions of dollars have been spent and fortunes made on this problem; you can easily find reams of material on nutrition, food, and weight management, and a diet-related book of one kind or another perpetually on the Top 10 bestseller list. It's amazing how many ways a basic fact of life like eating can be restructured and repackaged, then marketed over and over with no real results.

But this fact remains: When you consume more calories than your body needs for fuel, those calories get stored as fat, and to lose weight you have to restrict calories, increase activity, or, ideally, do a combination of both.

Yet who doesn't want to eat their cake and look like Cindy Crawford too?

The problem is when this doesn't work and the numbers on the scale creep up, you become a sitting duck for the diet and weight-loss industry. You don't have to be, especially since diets aren't a long-term solution. One thing that helps is to face the challenge of modern times.

As mentioned earlier, up until the Industrial Revolution, most people's lives revolved around getting food from the garden or the wild to their larders, pantries, ice-houses, and finally the dinner table. This task, and other basics of living, required enormous effort and physical activity. Simply put: Once upon a time people burned every day, as a matter of course, two or three times the calories used today.

Combined with this enormous calorie expenditure was the fact that the food people used to eat was much different from what ends up on our dinner tables today. Then, there weren't the prepackaged, highly refined, highly processed foods that we now have. So people used to eat mostly seasonal produce, whole grains, and farm-raised dairy and meat products; they tended to consume foods straight out of nature and naturally higher in fiber and nutrients and lower in calories.

Yes, my Grandpa Huber ate sausage and eggs and biscuits with gravy, but he also ate three or more vegetables and fruits at every meal. And he probably had those biscuits and gravy completely burned off by his morning labors alone. His lifestyle could afford those calories. Our lifestyles cannot.

The only sensible solution to our battle with the bulge is to combine compassion and realism toward ourselves with gradual adjustments to our food intake and physical activity. Imagine if you treated yourself with loving-kindness and self-respect instead of falling victim to the diet industry. Or if you chose the majority of your foods from unrefined, unprocessed sources. And what if you increased the amount of calories you burned daily by being more physically active?

The natural food choices that seemed so simple for my grandparents take effort in this day and age, but they can be made. It's all much simpler than any of us have been led to believe.

⤛∞⤜

Knowledge is the process of piling up facts.
Wisdom lies in their simplification.
MARTIN H. FISCHER

Keeping a record of what you eat is a wonderful tool whether you need to lose weight or not. I recommend that you block out a small section in your wellness journal and simply record everything you eat and drink for one week. The purpose here isn't to track calories or fat grams, but to focus on food groups. By recording what you eat for one week, you can see clearly—in your own handwriting—the food choices you make on a daily basis. These records are nothing to be ashamed of, and you aren't writing things down to beat up yourself. This is a tool for awareness and self-care. Now, here are the primary elements to track:

- Water—how much?
- Other beverages
- Food—type and general amounts
- Time of day
- Where you are (home, work, restaurant)
- Who you are with (family, friends, alone)
- How you basically feel (good, tired, upset)

The first thing I look at when clients have tracked their diets for one week is how much water they drink daily. In fact, I feel so strongly about the life-supporting, health-giving properties of water, I won't remark on any other area of the food diary until a client habitually starts drinking plenty of water.

———— ∞ ————

Chronic and persistently increasing dehydration is the root cause of almost all currently encountered major diseases of the human body.
F. BATMANGHELIDJ, M.D., IN *YOUR BODY'S MANY CRIES FOR WATER*

Most people have no idea how important water is to their health or how much water they need to be healthy, and though water is not on the Food Guide Pyramid, it should be. It's not only a true elixir of health, energy, and beauty, but next to air it's the element needed most for life. Since the body is made up of 60 percent to 70 percent water, no person can survive more than a few days without water. The American Dietetic Association even found that just a 2 percent water deficit can result in a 20 percent decline in strength.

That's why every day you need to replenish the 10 to 12 gallons of water that your every metabolic and physiological functions depend upon. If you're drinking under eight glasses of water a day, this is the first improvement you'll want to make. First, measure a generous eight ounces in a measuring cup and see what size glass that really requires. Try to drink a glass first thing in the morning, before breakfast if possible; keep track of your water intake in your wellness journal or Daytimer. By noon you'll want to be halfway to your goal. One caveat—you may want to accomplish the bulk of your water drinking by 6:00 P.M.—or else you'll be getting up in the middle of the night, not a preference of mine.

One easy way to make drinking water a habit is to drink a glass every time you make a pit stop. Yes, for a while you'll feel like you're constantly running to the bathroom, but in time your bladder will hold more fluid comfortably and process it more efficiently. (Be aware of the color of your urine throughout the day too. The goal is to get it pretty much colorless and clear.)

Other tips to make water drinking an easy habit: Try to drink a glass about 30 minutes before every meal, and if you're out somewhere and offered a beverage, always ask for water. Or fill a two-liter bottle with water first thing in the morning to drink by the end of the day. For those on-the-go, a .5-liter (or 16.9-ounce) bottle of water easily slips into your purse to drink, refilling it three times over the course of a day.

I've never worked with anyone who didn't feel a lot better after integrating regular water drinking into his or her life. There are proven reasons for this: Water is essential to your body's ability to metabolize fat, plus when drinking more water you'll notice less tendency to overeat, better digestion, and improved skin tone. My complexion improves tremendously when I drink eight to ten glasses of water consistently as opposed to five or six. You'll also reduce your tendency to retain water, since the body actually holds onto water when it's not getting enough.

Several of my clients have lost a few pounds by making this single dietary change. However, the biggest reason to make this a priority is

89

for good health. Water is truly one of nature's best medicines, and in the full spectrum of lifestyle change, this one's significant. Until you master this goal, you may be spending a lot of time semi-dehydrated.

There are different theories about what kind of water is best. I drink a combination of reverse-osmosis filtered water and lemon-lime flavored seltzer. I think there's ample evidence to support drinking filtered or pure spring water over tap water, most of the time. Yet I'd avoid splitting hairs on this. Find a reputable filtered water that tastes good to you and simply focus on the habit of drinking more water.

It is difficult to think anything but pleasant thoughts
while eating a homegrown tomato.
LEWIS GRIZZARD

If water is our elixir of health, fruits and vegetables are Mother Nature's best vitamin pills. So once the habit of good, steady water consumption is in place, my next focus with my clients' diets is increasing the amount of fruits and vegetables eaten each day. The current Food Guide Pyramid, which I consider a sensible resource, suggests eating two to four servings of fruit and three to five servings of vegetables every day. In the last few years the Surgeon General, U.S. Department of Health and Human Services, and National Cancer Institute have all recommended at least five servings of fruits and vegetables (combined) every day to reduce the risk of heart disease and cancer.

It's great that all these organizations are finally stressing the importance of produce in our diets, but it's sobering to realize only about 20 percent of Americans meet the five-a-day minimum.

With that in mind, the five-a-day recommendation, like meeting water requirements, is a powerful goal to achieve. And it's not only safe and reasonable, but advantageous to eat three to five servings of both fruits and vegetables every day (although diabetics should limit fruit servings according to the advice of their physicians). Increasing fruits and vegetables is a great example of your power of choice.

I've always found it to be much more productive to maximize the good stuff we should be eating, rather than focusing on all the things we know we should not. I also think serving sizes of fruits and vegetables, for the sake of increasing overall consumption, could be more generous. For now, however, I'll stay within the framework of the pyramid, which describes serving sizes as any of the following:

Vegetables
- $1/2$ cup chopped raw or cooked
- 1 cup raw leafy
- $3/4$ cup juice

Fruit
- one medium piece—like an apple or pear
- one melon wedge
- $1/2$ cup chopped, cooked or canned
- $1/4$ cup dried (like raisins)
- $3/4$ cup juice

Look through your food record and add up the number of fruits and vegetables you eat each day. Don't be depressed if you're often short of five servings. Instead, focus on the incredible payoff you'll get by making this one improvement. Look at the types of produce you eat as well as the quantity. Everyone tends to get in a food rut now and then, missing delicious opportunities for healthful variety. Now consider how you can infuse your diet with these potent, life-giving foods. Remember, by the power of this small choice, you can dramatically affect your weight, well-being, and longevity.

Breakfast is a great time to begin. Orange juice or half a grapefruit, then banana and other fruit (like peaches or berries) on your cereal gets in three servings before your day really starts. Choosing a piece of fruit as a snack between meals is a great habit, as is choosing fruit for dessert. Compare, for instance, the choice between a Snickers bar at 280 calories and a Granny Smith apple at 125 calories. The candy bar delivers

10 grams of fat and 1 gram of fiber, while the apple provides zero fat and 5 grams of fiber, putting you closer to the American Dietetic Association's recommendation of 20 grams of fiber a day. (Speaking as a woman with a stash of chocolate somewhere in the house at all times, the Snickers bar remains the more appealing choice to your tastebuds. But what if you reached for an apple every other time you crave candy?)

Vegetables take a little more planning to work into your meals. The dinner salad made with iceberg lettuce and pale, hard tomatoes—still served at many restaurants—barely counts as a serving. The piece of wilted lettuce or single slice of tomato on a fast-food burger doesn't really count at all. What you need to increase is the number of servings of vibrantly colored veggies! Deep greens, yellows, reds, and purples are all signs of potent nutrients. Spinach salads, salads made with green leaf, red leaf, or romaine lettuce are great, especially when you go light on the dressing. Broccoli, asparagus, yellow squashes (like acorn and butternut), cabbage, sweet potatoes, corn, and tomatoes are all wonderful foods that should cross our lips on a regular basis.

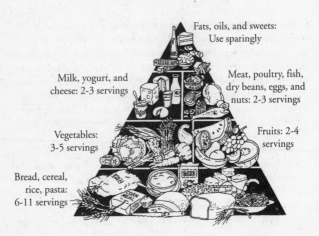

Fats, oils, and sweets:
Use sparingly

Milk, yogurt, and
cheese: 2-3 servings

Meat, poultry, fish,
dry beans, eggs, and
nuts: 2-3 servings

Vegetables:
3-5 servings

Fruits: 2-4
servings

Bread, cereal,
rice, pasta:
6-11 servings

Consider having a cup (or fist-size serving) of vegetables on a bed of rice or with a baked potato for lunch, most days of the week. At dinner, begin with a generous serving of raw salad chock full of things like scallions, red cabbage, shredded carrots, mushrooms, and bell pepper along with green leafy lettuce or spinach. Eat two or more side vegetables with whatever you're having for dinner—or consider making dinner nothing but vegetables a couple times a week. Believe me, there are enough kinds of vegetables available year-round to increase the variety of this fabulous food, even for the pickiest eater.

This much I can promise: As you start to munch on more fruits and vegetables, gradually increasing variety and quantity, you'll find yourself eating fewer processed and refined high-fat foods, your taste buds will begin to crave fresh produce straight from the good earth, and you'll be less enamored with the heavy, over-sauced and salted rich foods that have become the basis of the standard American diet. Your body will respond to fresh nutrients with heightened energy and easier digestion, and you'll probably even consume a greater volume of food with fewer calories and less fat, and feel more satisfied after meals. The gift you give your body, your immune system, and your digestive tract by implementing this one healthy eating habit is truly too great to measure.

As you add more fresh produce to your meals, by all means, give yourself some time to adjust. Add one serving of fruit and one serving of vegetable a day, and master that for a week before taking on more. Listen to your body's needs as you go along. While it's hard to go overboard on eating fresh produce, your body will let you know if you do. Cramping, bloating, or other digestive disturbances could indicate you're changing too much, too fast. So remember the goal of a diet adjustment is the same as for every suggestion in this book: Healthy choices need to work for you on a daily basis—for life.

The brown bread that Ma had made from the ground wheat was
very good. It had a fresh, nutty flavor that seemed almost
to take the place of butter.
LAURA INGALLS WILDER IN *THE LONG WINTER*

There's been a lot of press—good and bad—on carbohydrates the past several years. The media has alternately touted the virtues and evils of carbs depending on which diet is making the headline news. Since carbohydrates provide your most immediate source of accessible energy for physical and mental activity, it's important to know the whole story.

For instance, it's true that carbohydrates in the form of fruits, vegetables (especially legumes), and grains provide fuel for your body. And in the grain department the best choices are a variety of whole foods like oats, brown rice, whole wheat, whole grain breads, and enriched grain products that contain important B vitamins and folic acid.

However, most people don't get enough of these good carbohydrates, instead choosing too many refined flour products often containing sugar and fat. When you eat more carbohydrates than you need for fuel, they're stored as fat just like anything else. For example, bagels, muffins, noodles, crackers, and breads can be healthy choices, but be aware of the fat content in baked goods like muffins. Also fat-free baked goods like cookies and cakes often deliver an excess of sugar content and little nutritional value or fiber. This is why it's easy to gain weight on so-called high-carbohydrate diets. Technically, you may be choosing more carbs, but you might not be eating the complex, whole-grain ones you need for good nutrition and weight control.

But not only which carbohydrates you eat matter—it's how much that counts too. USDA and Health and Human Service nutritionists recommend this food group to provide 55 to 60 percent of your day's total intake. The Food Guide Pyramid recommends six to eleven servings of grains—bread, cereal, rice, and pasta—based on your calorie needs and activity, and three of these should be whole grain foods. Any of the following options on this list can help you see what counts as a serving of grains:

- one slice of bread
- one 7-inch tortilla
- $1/2$ cup cooked rice or pasta
- 1 ounce dry cereal
- half a bagel or English muffin

- six plain crackers
- two 4-inch pancakes
- three cups of air-popped popcorn

With this guide, do you see how it's entirely possible to eat most of a day's recommended six grain servings with just one of those jumbo bagels or muffins so popular today?

An easy step, then, toward weight control and improved nutrition is to take a closer look at the number and size of grain servings you eat on a given day. Refer to your food journal again, and note the choices you tend to make from the grain group. If you're like most people, you probably get plenty of bread, cereal, and pasta. But what other types of grains do you consume?

Do you ever eat rice, preferably brown rice? What about trying good old-fashioned oatmeal for breakfast? Or another cooked, whole grain cereal instead of the dry over-sugared, over-processed cereals that fill the cereal aisle? Do you ever eat kasha, millet, or polenta? These nutrient- and fiber-rich foods as old as time are easy to miss today. What about breads? Seek out a bakery that specializes in chewy, whole grain, European-style breads and try something new.

Look at the nutritional analysis of the bagels you eat, too, for how many servings of carbohydrates you're getting in one punch. You don't have to give up bagels, or anything for that matter. All foods fit into a healthy diet in moderation. Just consider increasing the diversity of your other grain choices, especially those high in fiber.

By increasing the number of whole grain foods you eat and adding choices like oats and rice to your menu, you can find new energy and even lose weight. Since the body responds favorably to even a little encouragement from the diverse and substantive whole, complex, unprocessed grain group, it's easy to understand how people survived for thousands of years on little more than grains.

So far you've seen the benefits of water consumption, eating three to five servings (minimum) of both fruits and vegetables a day, and choosing complex carbohydrates and diverse whole grains. Maintaining these three areas can positively affect health more than any other dietary change. As you move ahead with the top third of the pyramid, continue to approach food choices from the point of view of maximizing the good stuff.

———❧———

Hear, O Israel, and be careful to obey . . . that you may increase greatly in a land flowing with milk and honey . . .
DEUTERONOMY 6:3

It's easy to associate the word "milk" back to the very day you were born, since during the first months of life your mother's milk or a milk-like formula was all the nourishment you knew. Along with the milk came the sense of nurturing and care as you nursed. No wonder, then, that long after infancy milk and milk products are so often a source of comfort and satisfaction.

Think of the way you use milk and its by-products. *Milk and honey.* This is what I often drank just before bedtime during my stressful years at Juilliard. *Milk and cereal.* This was typical breakfast fare for our family when I was a little girl, and the best part of it was slurping the last dregs of milk and sugar from the bottom of the bowl. *Cookies and milk.* I frankly don't know how I would have survived my teenage years without the pleasure and comfort of retreating to my room after school to read a book, lying on the floor as I dipped my mom's wonderful peanut butter cookies in a tall glass of milk. *Creamy tapioca pudding . . . Mom's unbelievable banana cream pie covered with whipped cream . . .* no doubt you have good memories of scrumptious desserts like these as well.

Certainly, more Americans are enjoying more yogurt, cheese, butter, and ice cream than ever, although there's been a real shift in the perception of milk's health benefits. Dairy products used to occupy a higher place in the American diet when they were considered one of the four food groups. Today dairy appears in the upper third of the pyramid, and you're encouraged to consume more lowfat and nonfat milk products for weight control and good health, while limiting high-fat items like butter and cream. This is a good trend all in all, and I believe recommendations eventually may be to use dairy in your diet with even more restriction—perhaps like a condiment. After all, though milk and its by-products are a good source of calcium, protein, and B vitamins, they can be high in saturated fat, cholesterol, and calories. Also, milk is an animal product, so it doesn't qualify for being low-on-the-food-pyramid status.

How much dairy product should you be getting? Just two to three servings, and a serving is considered to be any of the following:

- 1 cup milk or yogurt
- 1 1/2–2 ounces hard cheese
- 2 ounces processed cheese
- 1/2 cup cottage cheese
- 1 cup frozen yogurt

Being a believer in moderation, I don't have a problem with these recommendations as long as the choices are lowfat and nonfat most of the time. Keep in mind, however, that even lowfat milk products can deliver a pretty high fat-gram punch. An easy way to assess the right amount without a scale or other measurement tool is to think of a serving of cheese as about the size of a pair of dice. That's probably smaller than what you've visualized in the past. The fact is increasing evidence shows that in societies and cultures where people consume a fraction of the dairy foods we do, there's a lower incidence of heart disease and cancer.

How many servings do you consume each day? Have you ever experimented with milk substitutes like soy- or rice-based milks?

I've known many people who began living dairy-free and believed this alone to improve their general well-being, clearing up everything from chronic digestive ailments and fatigue to skin problems and headaches.

Indeed, milk is a common source of food allergies and sensitivities; plenty of other foods—like vegetables, grains, beans, and raw seeds—can provide the nutrients you get from milk.

Again, I'm not pointing a finger at milk and saying, "This is a bad food." I don't think of any foods in terms of "good" or "bad," just in terms of how they maximize health. So if you enjoy your daily servings of milk products and you're careful about fat content, fine. Just be aware that dairy-free living is a viable option, with benefits. Your body can tell you if this is an option for you or not; it's important to acknowledge your own uniqueness with the foods best for you and the ones that are not.

Let the stoics say what they please, we do not eat for the good of living,
but because the meat is savory and the appetite is keen.
RALPH WALDO EMERSON

Most of the research on the standard American diet over the past thirty years points to the virtues of eating limited animal flesh. Every year that I live, animal sources of food take up less and less of my diet. I've embraced this mainly vegetarian diet for the last twenty-plus years and just eat a little chicken and fish when I feel the urge.

My interest in health foods and eating lower on the food chain actually started when I was sixteen. I spent a summer working on a cattle ranch outside of Billings, Montana, and experienced firsthand the reality of the beef industry: from the shaky steps of a newborn calf, and branding and vaccinating of a herd, to the sale of heifers and steers at the feed lot auctions, to the taste of a side of beef from a ranch-raised cow.

What struck me after leaving the ranch was the difference in the look, taste, and texture of farm-raised meat from that at the grocery store. Between the sale of a steer at an auction to its final destination—the plate of a consumer—something pretty wild happens to that animal product.

As I explored vegetarianism after that summer, the dangers of growth hormones and pesticide residues in meat resonated with me. I knew the grocery store beef had been through several stages of preparation for commercial sale because it didn't remotely resemble the beef I'd eaten on the ranch. The seed for vegetarianism was firmly planted before I turned twenty. Now, as more and more studies indicate the link between eating meat and our country's high incidences of heart disease, cancer, and other chronic disease, I'm doubly convinced that vegetarian sources of protein are nutritionally superior and better for us than meat.

However, if you're not ready to make meat-eating a thing of the past, at least consider a few adjustments. Treat a meat serving like a small side dish rather than the main course of your meal. Experiment several times a week with meals that instead of meat include tofu or beans.

The goal should be to meet those needs without exceeding them. Unfortunately, our culture encourages getting almost twice the protein you need on a daily basis. When your body gets too much protein, it puts a strain on your liver and kidneys—and what isn't used for tissue repair gets stored as fat.

How much is enough? You can determine your protein needs, based on your age and activity level (see chart on page 87). A serving is any of the following:

- $2^1/2$–3 ounces cooked meat, poultry, or fish
- 1 cup of cooked beans
- 2 to 3 eggs (use 1 yolk for every 2 eggs)
- $3/4$ cup tofu

An easy way to work with these guidelines is to remember a three-ounce portion of meat or fish is about the size of a cassette tape, considerably smaller than what's served at a restaurant or routinely eaten at the dinner table. In fact, a typical paperback book-sized slab of salmon fillet, chicken breast, or sirloin steak exceeds in a single serving the amount of protein you need for an entire day.

Also remember you can get protein from other parts of the food pyramid that are lower in fat and calories and higher in nutrients and fiber. For instance, the oatmeal I eat at breakfast supplies five grams of protein, the brown rice I eat at lunch counts for thirteen grams, and the broccoli I eat at dinner has another five grams. These foods are less processed and closer to the earth than a piece of meat and carry other benefits without chemicals or cholesterol.

The hero is not fed on sweets.
RALPH WALDO EMERSON

With all the controversy and hype about what to eat, it's easy to forget that food's meant to nourish and sustain, give pleasure, and bring together families and friends. By maximizing the lower two-thirds of the Food Guide Pyramid and drinking a lot of water, you can receive the full blessing and health benefits of a prudent and enjoyable diet. But at the very top of the pyramid is the category of fats, oils, and sweets, which are abundantly available and calorically dense—so this is a category of foods where it pays to choose carefully.

You probably already know the bottom line on fat—that it's higher in calories (nine per gram) than any other food whether it's in a solid form like butter, margarine, or lard; a liquid form like oil; or part of an animal, like skin on chicken or in beef. It's also recognized instantly by the body as something to be stored for later use, not burned easily like carbohydrates or used for tissue repair like protein. But did you know that you do need a small amount of fat in your diet to supply the fatty acids that help absorb the fat-soluble vitamins A, D, E, and K?

However, the common consensus in diet research is that you get more fat than you need, so you should limit your intake to no more than 30 percent of your daily calories. I encourage my clients to aim for 20 percent and celebrate actually netting around 25 percent. I'm not a real fan of calorie-counting, but here's an equation worth doing: One tablespoon of any kind of fat provides about 125 calories or 14 grams of fat. Let's say you need 2,000 calories a day and want to limit your fat to 20 percent. Simply multiply the calorie need (2,000) by 0.2 (20 percent) and divide by 9 (calories per gram); 2,000 x 0.2 = 400 ÷ 9 = 44 (rounded). Since a single tablespoon of butter or oil provides 14 grams, see how quickly fat grams add up?

It's important to remember that certain fats are healthier than others. The most healthful fats you consume are monosaturated. Olive oil, avocados, nut oils like walnut and grapeseed or flax oils, fish oils, and canola oils are the best sources. The downside of saturated fats from animal sources like dairy and meat is well known, so it's important to minimize these in your diet. Polyunsaturated fats like corn and peanut oil, margarines, and palm and coconut oils have been steadily looking less healthful as more research is done—I would avoid them. In fact, unless your doctor says otherwise, I would recommend using a small amount of butter over margarine, which contains hydrogenated (hardened) fat. I would avoid olestra, the new fat substitute, at all costs. We are all guinea pigs for food substitutes like olestra, saccharin, and aspartame—and I don't think our bodies know what to do with this stuff.

Sweets—my personal splurge of choice—frequently compound the calorie density of sugar with the calorie punch of fat. Muffins, cookies, cakes, pies—whatever gets your sweet tooth going—are fattening, mainly because of the combination of fat and sugar more than the preponderance of one or the other. Sugar is not an evil or poisonous food. It's just nutritionally empty with a high-calorie cost. Sweet foods can also be trigger foods that lead to out-of-control eating.

My rule of thumb follows the idea that moderation in the long run is healthier, gentler, and more realistic. If you really crave something, enjoy a moderate amount of it and move on. I'd rather eat a small portion of the real thing, like a freshly baked brownie or a dish of ice cream, than try to satisfy my craving with substitute foods I don't really like that much. By giving yourself permission to have whatever you want, as long as it's a reasonable quantity, you defuse a whole cycle of deprivation, obsession, and frustration, which sets in with rigid controls. In this sense you can have your cake and eat it too—as long as it's not with every meal every day.

Live in each season as it passes; breathe air, drink the drink, taste the fruit, and resign yourself to the influences of each. Let them be your only diet drink and botanical medicines.

HENRY DAVID THOREAU IN HIS JOURNALS, ENTRY FOR AUGUST 23, 1853

Can you imagine a life without food? What a bleak existence it would be in absence of the ritual of eating. Because as important as the food choices are that you make—and they're important—the way you eat impacts your health just as much.

Yet one of the great tragedies in our culture is how we're losing the art of enjoying the simplest things in life. People today are so frantic and busy working and consuming that it's almost been forgotten how to just be. You've probably experienced this, frequently eating on the run, being pushed for time, distracted by the television, and without the fellowship of others. It makes no sense to maximize your diet without maximizing your enjoyment of it too.

So when, where, and how happily do you experience the ritual of eating? Observe these things in your wellness journal. Then consider the following suggestions to return the ritual of eating to a place of grace and comfort in your daily life:

- **Take time to eat, seated at a table or at least in a chair, undistracted by the television and the hustle and bustle of life.** Make your environment as gracious and inviting as possible. I love reading while I eat—which is not recommended by weight-loss experts—but as long as it doesn't lead to overeating, I don't have a problem with reading a good book or article while enjoying a meal.
- **Give thanks before you start.**
- **Put your fork down and chew each bite thoroughly and swallow before picking up the utensil again.** Don't eat anything you don't enjoy—save the calories for something you love.
- **Notice periodically if you feel full so you don't eat more than your body needs.** Keep in mind that satiety—the feeling of fullness—doesn't transmit instantly from the stomach to the brain. It takes about twenty minutes to register.
- **Remember to take time to savor the ritual as much as the food and to breathe deeply while you eat.** Breathing connects you with your body and how you really feel, but it takes a deliberate effort to get beyond shallow breathing to deeper breaths. If you're eating with someone else, take time to talk—and listen— as the communion shared when breaking bread with one

another is a blessing. Folding your hands in your lap between bites is another way to be less rushed. You may find you can leave the table completely satisfied with less food than you think, when you just take your time.

- **Refuse to eat while driving the car or on the run.** This is a destructive habit and a sad commentary on today's lives. If you don't have time to sit for five minutes to eat an apple or half of a sandwich, even on the busiest day, you need to look at the choices you're making in other areas of your life. Any change you make to return serenity and civility to this aspect of your life will be rewarded tenfold. I've eaten frantically and I've eaten peacefully, and nothing could send me back to frantic eating again. The way you treat yourself with food is a reflection of how you value your life and health.

Finally, as you put everything on diet and water together, remember to keep food simple and gentle. Eating healthful foods is only a part of being well, as the most devoted macrobiotic enthusiast can still suffer a serious disease. You can make this part of your wellness a priority, however, without making it an obsession. It's better to sit down as a guest at someone's table and enjoy a little bit of everything than to mentally review your fruit servings for that day.

The Power of Choice

Things you can do every day to impact your well-being

- **You're likely to drink more when it tastes good.** For me, water becomes much more palatable with a squeeze of lemon or lime. I keep at least one fresh lemon in my refrigerator at all times for this purpose.

- **Invest in a juicer.** Fresh vegetable and fruit juice tastes delicious and is good for you. I recommend buying a professional model like the Waring Professional Juice Extractor or the Champion Juicer. For you skeptics, try a combination of carrot, apple, and ginger. It's tasty, foamy, and packed with nutrients. This is also an economical way to use up produce that otherwise gets thrown away.

- **Eat what you want, but be realistic about the consequences by taking advantage of the Nutrition Facts food analysis on packaged foods.** Avoid foods that have more than five grams of fat per serving; three grams and under is even better. Also, check what constitutes one serving for that food product. Is it a reasonable amount, or would you eat twice that much as a typical serving? For instance, whoever ate just one-half cup of ice cream or just two teaspoons of grated cheese?

- **Use this easy way to recognize serving sizes without messing with a food scale or measuring cups.** One ounce of meat or cheese is about the size of a matchbox. A three-ounce serving of fish, chicken, or meat is the size of a cassette tape. Eight ounces of meat (way too much for one serving) looks like a small paperback book. A cup of pasta, rice, or potatoes is about the size of your fist; a cup of leafy salad is slightly larger. Don't confuse typical restaurant portions for reasonable servings, as they're generally much larger and more calorie dense than anyone would like to acknowledge.

- **Think of ways to celebrate your meals.** Place a single flower in a bud vase on the table or light a candle to create a peaceful atmosphere. Surround yourself with beauty and grace, especially at mealtimes.

- **It's much more difficult to indulge in high-fat, high-calorie food if you don't buy it to begin with;** it's also much easier to eat low on the food chain when appealing fruits, vegetables, and grains are readily available. Keep your refrigerator stocked with good choices. If you do splurge on a rich treat, do it with gusto, eat it slowly, and enjoy everything about it without any guilt.

- **Find a market that specializes in great, fresh produce.** We have one in Nashville called the Produce Place, where I do my shopping on Saturday mornings and am always inspired by the bins of great fruits and vegetables. I find that I make better choices when not distracted by the millions of things on the shelves of regular supermarkets. Treat your food shopping with discernment and make this part of the process of eating as enjoyable as possible.

- **Know that fat-free foods are not all they're cracked up to be.** Fat-free salad dressings, cheeses, and the like are generally filled with a lot of unpronounceable ingredients that don't resemble food. I find lowfat versions to be so much more tasty and satisfying, they're worth the additional calories.

- **Another way to approach calorie control naturally is to dilute the real thing.** I pour one-half bottle of my favorite salad dressing (Newman's Own Oil & Vinegar) into a jar for later use and add balsamic vinegar and water to the original bottle. This way I enjoy the flavor of the real thing while consuming half the calories. I find reduced-fat rather than nonfat baked items to be superior as well. When all the fat is removed from baked goods, the sugar content goes way up in an effort to make them taste good. Satisfy your craving with either the real thing or a reduced-fat version, and you'll probably come out ahead.

- **Check labels for ingredients.** Look for products that have high-quality, lowfat, low sugar ingredients and try to avoid those with mysterious words you can't pronounce.

- **Read *Eating Well, Living Well: When You Can't Diet Anymore*** by Glenn A. Gaesser, Ph.D., and Karin Kratina, M.A., R.D. Published by the Wheat Foods Council, this is one of the best resources on healthy eating I've ever found and includes an excellent review of the popular fad diets. To order online, log onto www.wheatfoods.org, call (303) 840-8787, or write for information to the Wheat Foods Council, 10841 S. Crossroads Drive, Suite 105, Parker, CO 80138.

Five

Balance

By the seventh day God had finished
the work he had been doing;
so on the seventh day he rested
from all his work. And God blessed
the seventh day and made it holy,
because on it he rested from all the
work of creating that he had done.

GENESIS 2:2–3

One of the great ironies of our time is that people expend enormous amounts of energy to buy and decorate their homes, but rarely take the time to enjoy them. What about you?

Before you answer, I want you to try something. Turn off the ringer on your phone. Go into the kitchen and fix yourself something to drink—a cup of tea, hot chocolate, or glass of sparkling water with lemon. Take it to your favorite room in the house, light a scented candle, and place it near your comfiest spot. Take off your shoes, enjoy the feel of curling up, the glow of the candle, and taste of your beverage. Sit with this feeling for a moment. Breathe in the quiet and notice what you love about this spot, this room. What makes it special to you? Why is it your favorite place in the house?

As you sit, breathe, and reflect, let your eyes travel to the pictures on the walls, the window dressings, and furniture around you. As I write this, my eyes rest on a beautifully framed poster from a blue-grass festival I played with John Hartford in Telluride, Colorado, more than ten years ago. I can still be there in my mind from the memories of that poster alone. What do you notice about the other things in your surroundings that give you pleasure? Is it the color of the paint on the walls or the way the light comes through the windows? Is there a beautiful plant you enjoy or a favorite vase displayed? I have a collection of teacups in my sitting room—some that I've bought over the years and a cherished set from Grandma Huber, which was a gift for my hope chest. In my quiet moments I enjoy picking up some of the cups. I run my fingers over the fine china, admire the designs, and think of Grandma's legacy of love and strength. Whatever surrounds you, take a moment to enjoy it. Bask in the peace and contentment that accompany a few minutes of silence and rest.

Now take a moment to reflect on the recent weeks and months of your life. Think about all the work you've done. Make a mental list of all the energies you expend as you go through a typical day. Does racing across town, hustling and bustling at work, getting the kids to school, stopping at the grocery store, cleaning the house, paying bills, intervening in catastrophes, taking care of a sick or elderly loved one, or just being available to everyone sound familiar? Until now, when's the last time you took time out from the countless tasks in your life to sit down and enjoy quiet in your home?

If it's been a long time ago or you can't really remember a quiet time like this, you're not alone. Balance and rest from labor can be foreign concepts in today's culture. These basic human needs have been so abused and neglected in our fast-paced world that our whole culture cries out for relief from this attack on the soul.

Work, sometimes very hard work, is a fact of life for most people— and always has been. My grandparents labored from dawn to dusk most of their days. But on Sundays they rested—really rested. On Saturdays, Grandma Huber did all the Sunday meal preparation, except for putting food in the oven, to avoid laboring on the Sabbath. Likewise, Grandpa Huber would let crops get ruined in the rain, rather than work on the day of rest. Together, they always went to church and Sunday school and spent the rest of the day at leisure.

On their summer days, there might be a picnic in the park, or men and women would visit and maybe play a game of horseshoes or go for a walk by the lake. No movies, no shopping, no catching up on office work or sitting in front of the TV for sporting events—just simple, enjoyable rest.

But beyond this gracefulness of Sundays, my grandparents enjoyed a measure of serenity each day of the week too. They had one phone hanging on the kitchen wall, and it was a party line, so conversations were short. As my mom put it: You didn't say anything on the phone that you didn't want everyone to know. Their phone was a link to the outside world, not an instrument of invasion like it is today. No one

109

called to sign you up for another credit card or to get you to renew your magazine subscription; everyone respected basic courtesies like the right to privacy. Stress and commercialism had not yet invaded the fabric of daily life.

In fact, my grandparents had a radio in their home but no TV. They listened to nightly broadcasts—from news and stories to music and plays—while relaxing in rocking chairs (my grandma, no doubt, with a crochet project in her lap). They heard the news without the graphic, violent pictures we witness on television today. They enjoyed the stories and plays, using their imaginations to see the different vignettes. Reading and playing games like Chinese checkers or canasta were more often the means of entertainment, with nothing more than the sound of the wind rustling the leaves outside. Peace and quiet were woven into each day, no matter how hectic or grueling the day had been.

Most of us don't realize how deeply we need this kind of graceful balance on a daily basis. We also don't realize just how depleted our resources are until a crisis hits. Our culture screams at us constantly to work more, earn more, do more, spend more—and we respond by expecting more of ourselves. The problem is most of us are already wrung dry. Insomnia, fatigue, autoimmune diseases, and headaches plague us while modern life continues its refrain: Do, get, be.

People used to have time to live and enjoy themselves, but there is no time anymore for anything but work, work, work.
LAURA INGALLS WILDER FROM *WORDS FROM A FEARLESS HEART*

Discovering that you need balance just as you need food and air can be tricky. For limited amounts of time you can produce work on an unbelievable scale without honoring your need for rest, and our culture applauds this. After all, it looks really good from the outside to work tirelessly, do a lot, stay busy, and achieve the unachievable.

But along the way more and more people are pushed to the edge of crisis and chaos. I not only see this with my clients, I also see it as I go to the store, the post office, and the bank. I see it in the faces of fatigued and burned-out workers, in the drooping shoulders of exhausted mothers, and in the frantic actions of drivers speeding from one destination to another with cell phones glued to their ears. Exhaustion trickles into people of all ages and socioeconomic backgrounds. Burnout is relentless, progressive, and ultimately destructive. Whenever personal value is determined by what you do, how much you earn, how hard you work, and how much you own, your life becomes meaningless.

In fact, this mind-set is a trap—one we all fall into sooner or later. I fell into it for a longer time than I care to admit. I thought if I just did a little more, worked a little harder, and achieved a higher standard, I'd be a better person. I came by this honestly enough. Most people do. After all, this is what's glorified in our culture. We don't read stories about people who sleep ten hours a night. We read about high achievers who get by on five. We don't hear about the person who has won a poetry contest. We hear about the star with a No. 1 hit song and a part in a movie at the same time. We're not exposed to people with inspiring personal triumphs like recovering from an accident to walk normally again. We're exposed to how great the celebrity of the month looks in the latest movie. Our culture offers a tempting and flashy yardstick to measure our individual accomplishments—and it pulls us out of balance.

The only antidote for this cultural disease—and it is a disease—is a return to balance. Not the illusion of balance, but the reality of it. Eating the right foods and getting regular exercise are instrumental to a long and healthy life. But also essential, if not even more important, are rest and play, emotional and spiritual wellness, and your relationships to others.

To put this concept of balance in perspective, imagine looking through the lens of a kaleidoscope. Hold it up to the light and you see an explosion of color, patterns, and pieces of different shapes and sizes. As you turn the kaleidoscope, the pieces and colors take on a life of their own, creating a million different stained glass windows, sometimes crammed with color, other times delicately spaced. At a certain angle the cool colors of green, blue, and gray register; turn ever so slightly and the hot hues of red, purple and yellow burst through.

111

The colors and patterns constantly change, and I'm sure you would agree they're beautiful.

Except that you may never know such symmetry, your life is like that changing kaleidoscope. The vibrant colors and shifting patterns represent the diverse parts, and balance is the flow of time and attention you give all the pieces, nurturing your whole person and treating yourself with respect. You must guard against the cultural tendency of living your life drenched in just one color.

To take this one step further, leaf back through the pages of your calendar or appointment book. Take four or five highlighter pens of different hues and choose a typical week to color code your life. Use one color to highlight the time you spent at work, another for physical activity and recreation, a third for time you spent with the people you love, and a fourth on the hours you spent in spiritual reflection.

What do you see? A healthy balance will resemble the rainbow—some quiet time every day (maybe more on Sundays), a work day that includes a relaxed lunch with a friend or walk in the park, evenings that include family time and self-care, and regular periods of physical activity. But when you look at your life in living color, it's difficult to deny the real picture—and for many women today it may not be so rainbow-like.

See the importance of this exercise? The colors allow you to see your schedule and lifestyle for what it is—and the colors don't lie. They do provide you with the choice to make adjustments to achieve a better balance. This won't happen all at once but rather in a series of manageable and enjoyable steps. Be prepared for change, however, because integrating balance feels so good and is so satisfying you won't be able to step back ever again.

My venture into balance and rest has been a series of steps—some small, some large, sometimes forward two and back one. This hasn't been a small feat. "Working, doing, achieving" was my mantra from my childhood. Coming from a musical family with competition among my sisters—and being very aware of my status as the eldest—I learned to aim high, work tirelessly, and never be satisfied with my achievements. I learned to compartmentalize my time and bury myself in work, projects, lists, and goals. I learned how to be disciplined, organized, efficient, and busy.

What I didn't learn, and my self cried for as I reached my thirties, was how to rest, relax, and take care of my own needs. I was exhausted, depressed, empty, and incapable of spontaneity. No matter what I achieved or how much money I'd earned, it wasn't enough to fill the part of me that just wanted to rest awhile.

Progress came in a series of plateaus. First I learned to carve out time in a day to just sit quietly. Then I found that simple things could help wind me down: lighting candles, listening to soothing instrumental music, lingering in uninterrupted bubble baths, the occasional massage. I learned that eight hours of sound sleep at night was non-negotiable if I wanted to enjoy any quality in my days. Eventually I began to enjoy recreational activities on the weekends instead of always tackling housework or squeezing in another session with a client. It was a major breakthrough to spend time with my husband or friends instead of saying, "Sorry, I don't have enough time to do that."

My work with clients also affirmed the importance of balance. The one-on-one process of a trainer with a client crosses the boundaries of most professions, and without any inappropriateness a person's whole life could be opened to the continuum of fitness training and lifestyle counseling.

Here is how one of my clients experienced this. Barbara, a lawyer, wife, and mom of one young child, had signed up for a handful of sessions. We'd sometimes meet during her lunch hour at a studio where I worked. One day she came in dressed for exercise but very distracted. She'd been up most of the night with her son, left the house on a tense note with her husband, and faced a looming work deadline at the office. We'd barely done a few warm-up exercises when she burst into tears. She was physically and emotionally exhausted, and this hour that she'd set aside for exercise was her first outlet to express her fears and frustrations.

We ended up doing some gentle stretches and releases for her tight, stressed-out body while the tears continued to flow. By the end of the session I was massaging her hands and just listening to the stream of

113

her concerns. She left feeling much better and relieved of at least one crucial layer of stress. We both agreed that her priority for self-care might be to keep a counseling or massage appointment once a week instead of an exercise session.

Several months later I ran into Barbara at the grocery store, and she looked like a different person. She'd made some changes in her life to accommodate her family, including a lighter workload and more help from her husband. In the process Barbara discovered a radiance and renewed enthusiasm that allowed her to enjoy the rewards of a more restful, balanced lifestyle.

I'm still in that process of honoring my need for balance, and it's an ongoing challenge because I love to work. But the rewards of doing life differently are so great, I cannot imagine ever going back to the brutal pace I used to keep. With each step toward self-care and balance, I've felt a layer of the endless agenda peel off my body and soul.

One must liberate oneself . . . from complexities, from taking one's fate too much to heart, before being able to rejoice simply because one is alive and among the living.
CZESLAW MILOSZ

Finding a flow of balance in your lifestyle is a subtle art, because balance doesn't necessarily mean smooth sailing or having and doing it all. Living in balance is a shift you make—and you're the only one who can make it. This shift takes you from doing to being, from wanting to enjoying what you already have, from overextending to nurturing, and from chasing illusions to standing still and listening. These shifts won't be initiated or even understood by the world around you, but your families and friends will benefit—and so will you.

Eventually your need for balance hits you in the face. It's not as tangible and obvious as changing your diet or increasing physical activity. First it tugs and pulls on your heart like a child grabbing a mother's skirt for attention. Or it creeps up on you like a car you've passed racing through traffic in the fast lane. You zoomed past that car several blocks ago, then notice it just got to the stop light at the same time you did. You continue to drive in the fast lane because you're sure it's the shortest distance between two points, but you keep looking at that other car. You're intrigued with doing life differently, but aren't sure you want to change lanes.

Then you get a wake-up call. Your body gets sick with a flu that no antibiotic can touch. Or maybe a loved one dies unexpectedly and you have to bear the grief of their passing and all the occasions you didn't have time to share with them. Or you discover your marriage is not the Rock of Gibraltar you assumed, or that one of your kids is experimenting with drugs. You can't remember the last time you received a letter in the mail, then realize you haven't written a letter in years. Small annoyances that shouldn't bother you suddenly send you into a rage. Tears of frustration and fatigue lurk continually just below the surface.

You realize, then, you've bought into the great lie of our culture to have and do it all. Most of us give this dream a larger portion of ourselves and our lives than we should. The lucky ones are those who see through the lie and make the shift sooner than later. I'm immensely grateful for starting to shift while still in my thirties, but every day I'm reminded of how easy it is to stay in that fast lane a little longer, because the illusion of having and doing it all is so intoxicating.

Sometimes the grim, dark moments of life can lead to a better place. The year I began writing this book had its share of such moments. In the space of three months, I lost a dear uncle who had been in declining health, heard of the sudden and shocking death of a former fiancé, and learned that my favorite aunt had been diagnosed with lymphoma.

Up to this time I'd been satisfied with my progress toward a more balanced existence. I was even planning to marry John. Although I was planning our wedding, I began feeling less joy over that event than I should have, and I found myself frequently overwhelmed with work and easily fatigued.

During one premarital counseling session, our therapist leaned toward me and said, "Ruth, you're too young and too healthy to be

115

this tired all the time. You must find a way to clear your plate and lighten your load."

This advice came at the time when I was keenly aware of how fleeting life is. I decided I didn't want to spend one more day of it too busy or too tired. The year continued to unfold with more stresses and challenges than I'd ever seen or hope to again, but the way I navigated through it was different. My priorities were in order. My ability to delegate took a giant step forward. I rested in my faith with a new degree of surrender. Life became much sweeter, and I drank deeply of it with gratitude for both the good times and the sad.

Perhaps the greatest gift in this process came from having to say good-bye to people I loved. I know that sounds strange—death isn't a subject most people want to dwell on, but facing the reality of it can be enormously freeing. All of us live just a heartbeat away from death. Like a laser, knowing this can cut through the things that don't matter.

That became clear in Nashville when Gwen, a lovely, dark-haired woman in the prime of her life—a gifted artist and singer, loved by everyone who met her, died in a freak accident while attending an art workshop in California. The music and art worlds came together in a memorial service to celebrate her unique life, and to mourn her passing. Friends and colleagues sang or played beautiful tributes and voiced eloquent remembrances, and an exhibit of Gwen's own paintings served as a poignant testament to a life well lived. As the service unfolded, I was struck by how many lives Gwen had touched. I saw friends connect in sorrow and affection, wives and husbands touch each other's arms with renewed appreciation, and heard stories of faith and love. The way Gwen lived her full and varied life cut a unique swath through time, people, and places.

Ultimately, a life with balance is to be like Gwen's: lived to the fullest with energy and enthusiasm, rich with human experiences and connections to other people; full of moments that seem to freeze time, shared glances that contain a conversation without words, experiences so compelling that the heart feels too big for the body—and the body seems too small for all the feelings. A life in balance is not marked by monetary wealth, possessions, or achievements. Instead it's a life that feels the full spectrum of joy and sorrow. It's raw and terrible at times, and exultant at others, but never boring, unsatisfying, or numb.

—◦◦◦—

A man can only do what he can do. But if he does that each day he can sleep at night and do it again the next day.
ALBERT SCHWEITZER

So how do you begin to shift into this life of balance? With good rest, for one thing. But you wouldn't guess that from the frantic pace of the modern American lifestyle. Today some 87 million Americans have trouble sleeping, and we're sleeping two hours less per night than our grandparents did and their parents at the turn of the century. This sleep deprivation has become not only a cultural epidemic, but both debilitating and deadly.

Many factors encourage and contribute to the problem. As the demands and expectations of the technological age increased, so has the tendency to use sleep time to get more done—thinking it will also help you get ahead. It doesn't help that there are so many resources for distractions and entertainment: Electricity provides artificial light to extend the waking hours. Phones, fax machines, computers, and televisions provide activity to tap into, log onto, or watch 24 hours a day. The stress and stimulation of modern-day life also encourages sleeplessness when your head finally does hit the pillow. You're so wound up from your day, you can't get relief during the night even if you're totally exhausted.

I know the fatigue that follows a poor night's sleep as I had regular bouts of insomnia during certain phases of my musical career. One of the greatest pleasures, not to mention achievements, of my life has been returning to a natural, easy sleep. But this evolved only when I started listening to my body's needs and treating bedtime with respect—simply knowing I needed more rest wasn't enough. After all, it's conceivable for a person to get plenty of sleep and still be out of balance. But it's impossible to live a life with balance and not honor one's individual need for sleep.

117

That's because with sleep you can see how all the elements of wellness work together. Sleep and water top the list of essential elements to wellness, and when you shortchange your sleep needs, the rest of your good health intentions tumble like dominoes: You become too tired to exercise and more likely to indulge in caffeine and sugar for a quick pickup. Ongoing sleep deprivation can make you more susceptible to colds and illnesses, chronic fatigue, burnout, and depression. This level of exhaustion gets into its own holding pattern and can last for years! Finally you get sick and tired of being sick and tired, but you're too tired to do anything about it.

The flip side is that when you feel rested from sufficient sleep, you're more apt to take care of yourself, have the energy to exercise, and sleep better from all that physical activity. That combination helps you make better food choices, which fuels your body's ability to function at a higher level, and as your quality of life improves, you're less drawn to unhealthy living habits.

So how do you begin to improve your chances of a good night's sleep? First, listen to what your body needs to determine the best time for sleep and the amount needed. Remember that every person is a creature of habit and rhythm. Since the beginning of time human beings have lived in cycles that naturally recognize day and night, as well as the four seasons (and it's only in the past century that these behaviors have blurred the distinctions, thanks to technology). For instance, it's natural to be awake and alert during the daylight hours, and natural to want rest and sleep as the sun goes down and night falls. When you disrupt these rhythms by staying up too late, frequently changing time zones, or getting up at different times, your body gets thrown out of rhythm, confused, and your sleep suffers.

Beyond the natural rhythms of day, night, and season, there's also an individual rhythm that governs the body clock. Some people are night owls who thrive staying up late and sleeping late. Others (like me) turn into pumpkins around 9:00 P.M. but love getting up early.

Create a routine that's right for you and consistent night after night. From time to time, travel, shift changes at work, children who need attention in the middle of the night, or other stressful life experiences will annihilate sleep. In these situations, other forms of self-care can temporarily take up the slack. For me, it helps to be vigilant to drink more water and eat well when professional obligations or a tough training schedule requires I start very early every morning of the week. At times like these I'll also try to make and drink juice more often and take every opportunity I can to sit quietly and breathe deeply.

Another help for better sleep is to begin following calming rituals for bedtime. It's unrealistic, after all, to expect your body and mind to simply turn off at the end of a hectic day and give you the rest you need to hit the ground running come morning. Just as you benefit from eating slowly in a serene setting, your sleep is more natural and easy if you allow wind-down time at the end of every day. Part of the winding-down process is to eat dinner early enough to let it digest and settle, and not to eat too much at the evening meal. Also avoid exposure to violent or upsetting television programs just before bed.

Your body will respond well to consistency with calming rituals for bedtime. Sleep specialists encourage this relaxing routine at bedtime: Take a bath, sip a calming (and decaffeinated) beverage, and read for 15 minutes or write in a journal.

I find that turning the lights down low in the evening helps ease me into sleep mode, and the hour before bedtime I avoid stressful paperwork and look for ways to quiet things in the house—meaning no TV, loud music, or planned phone conversations. Right before I turn in, I like to sit on the kitchen floor with my dogs, scratch them on the head, and talk to them for a while. Then I read for a short time before turning out the light. Over the years I've developed another habit as my head hits the pillow, and it's probably contributed more to my easy sleep routine than anything else: As I close my eyes and settle in I utter a few words of prayer, thank God for the day, and release my concerns to his great wisdom. I'm usually fast asleep within 10 minutes.

On weekends that follow a tough week, I've learned to build in extra tranquility and rest. Knowing that relief is around the corner helps me stay focused and relaxed in the face of sleep challenges.

Perhaps the best tool I've discovered over the years is learning to relax about the amount of sleep I'm not getting. Anyone who's ever spent a night tossing and turning knows that feeling of watching the clock relentlessly advance as the mind refuses to slumber. The key here is not to panic, which just feeds the cycle, or to keep checking the clock, which is an exercise in futility.

On these nights—and we all have them—focus on resting your physical body as much as possible, even if your mind is in a whirl. First, get as comfortable as you can in your bed. Adjust the room temperature if you need to, and the coverings so you're not too hot or too cold. If necessary, cushion your body with extra pillows. When sleeping on my side, I've found that an extra pillow under the top leg positions my back properly and makes me feel better. Once you've settled into a good position, focus on enjoying the sensation of being comfortable. Concentrate on deepening and slowing your breath and observe this breathing cycle. Since usually it's the mind that keeps you awake on nights like this, occupy your thoughts with something as innocuous as breathing. This takes some practice, but you'll soon find the ideas racing around your head may melt into a dreamy state enough to let you sleep. The best thing about this technique is, it builds sleep confidence without the use of drugs.

The sleep that comes with drugs is not as refreshing as natural sleep anyway. So while sleeping pills are available to help on rare occasions, I don't recommend them. In fact, though it can sometimes be more important to get needed rest than to hold out for natural sleep, this is not often. I'd encourage infrequent use of sleep medication and only under the supervision of a doctor.

Sanctuary

In a society that batters more than it nurtures, every person needs sanctuary or, depending on the word you prefer, solitude, a haven or an oasis. In my quest for balance I've learned to experience sanctuary in many places over the course of every day: the quiet of the early morning hours before anyone is up in our house, the stillness at the end of the day as I lower the shades and turn down the lights, the powerful silence during the early service at church that helps me imagine "the peace that passes all understanding," the tranquil trail through the woods where I walk.

Perhaps the most important place to feel sanctuary, though, is at home. Every person needs this place of rest from the chaos of the world—a place to build up the reserve to face whatever life is going to bring next, and that feeds the soul and offers a respite from the exhausting pace of modern life.

The easiest way to create this place at home is to increase opportunities for silence. Most households can accomplish this by simply turning off the TV, or at least seriously limiting its roar. (As you've probably guessed by now, I can't say enough about TV-free living.) Contrary to how it's perceived culturally, watching television does not relax the mind or body. Instead the constant chatter and babble wears you down without you realizing it, and programming that's increasingly suggestive and violent can attack and invade your soul.

You can open a wonderful window of silence by simply trying TV-free living for one week. You're sure to see your household calm down. Then, when the week is over, be willing to limit what you watch and how. For instance, why not tape the shows you really enjoy and zap through the commercials? You'll save yourself time and avoid the audibly louder blare of advertising, much of which can insult your intelligence.

Another way to cut down on intrusive noise is to keep civilized hours with the telephone, fax machine, and computer or e-mail. With few exceptions I won't answer the phone during dinner, allowing interruptions to this important time for my husband and me to catch up on our respective days. Instead I'll let my answering machine pick up any messages, and I'll return those calls after dinner. Then at 8:30 the phone is off for the night.

Why not let your answering machine or voice mail work for you as much as possible? As a result you can buffer your important time for reflection or connection with family and friends from the rat race outside.

Even if you have a home office, you can preserve your sense of sanctuary. Set limits on the hours you'll spend in front of the computer. Keep fax machines, computers, and other home office equipment out of the living room, kitchen, and bedroom—areas you need for restfulness and pleasure, not constant reminders of work.

Now think about beautifying your surroundings. This doesn't mean acquiring new things. I've worked in the homes of the very wealthy and of clients who live on a budget, and some of the most inspiring and graceful examples I've ever seen of hearth and home have been in the latter. That's because a home that's clean and uncluttered has a measure of peace that transcends expensive furnishings. The scent of freshly laundered bed coverings, sofa slipcovers, and bathroom towels is pleasant and uplifts, regardless of how worn or old; freshly picked flowers in a fruit jar can brighten any room, and the light of a candle can soften the plainest surroundings.

The point is you don't need money to heighten the pleasure and comfort you feel in your home—everyone is on the same playing field of potential. I'm as excited as the next person about redecorating and home improvement. However, as my husband and I wait for the right time to add on to our small one-bathroom house, we've learned to bask in the grace of all that we have. Much of that's come from a commitment to order, keeping things reasonably clean when and where we can, and making the most of simple opportunities for beauty: candles, flowers, a bowl of fruit on the kitchen counter, an old picture reframed, a fresh coat of paint across old walls. The result: Small investments—maybe just a little time and some imagination—really can add up to a peace that's priceless in creating sanctuary.

We are always doing something . . . talking, reading, listening to the radio, planning what next. The mind is kept naggingly busy on some easy, unimportant, external thing all day.
BRENDA UELAND FROM *IF YOU WANT TO WRITE*

Have you mastered the art of "multi-tasking"? You know what I mean—doing more than one thing at the same time, like applying your makeup in the car on the way to work, doing dishes while talking on the phone, making beds while you brush your teeth, or throwing a load of laundry into the wash while a pot is boiling over on the stove?

Then stop! This behavior, while tempting, is ultimately counterproductive to a balanced life. Doing two or three things simultaneously does not make you a better person. It makes you crazy. Plus, more often than not, your efforts to get ahead or be efficient in this manner lead you to miscalculations and accidents.

Instead, mindfulness—which is an integral part of balance—can free, relax, fulfill, and nurture you. Mindfulness is the art of focusing on where you are and what you're doing at the moment you're there and doing it; it's the exact opposite of trying to accomplish several things at once.

One of our greatest challenges to practicing mindfulness is resisting the pull of this culture to constantly reach for things you don't have at the expense of what you do. The problem with constantly striving for more—and most everyone gets caught up in this one way or another—is that it focuses on the destination rather than the path. Life is not about reaching goals. It's about the process of being on a meaningful path. The only moment you can ever truly have to celebrate or enjoy is the one that you're in. The simple and even the mundane is worthy of celebration because it's a part of real life, and life is precious.

The most basic practice of mindfulness is just sitting and being still. Remember trying this, sitting in your favorite room of the house, at the beginning of this chapter? Beyond this, there are many ways to be mindful. Washing the dishes, wiping off the kitchen counters, and setting a table just right are opportunities for mindfulness. Doing each thing with awareness to detail, without distraction or haste, brings beauty to simple tasks. It's a gift to yourself, and it enriches the lives you touch. It's also a reflection of how much you respect life, yourself, and others.

Sometimes you have opportunities to really soak in an experience but miss out on it because your mind is engaged elsewhere. An example of this for me is mentally reviewing my to-do list while I'm out running on a beautiful day. This is a psychosis of sorts—and doesn't get me any farther ahead, just wastes a beautiful day. Notice when and how you indulge in this behavior. Can you go to a concert or a movie and really be there for the whole thing? Or do you find your mind reviewing lists and preparing for future events while your body sits at the theater? Be aware of this when it happens and pull yourself back into the present. Ask yourself: "What can I possibly gain by separating my mind from where I am?" More importantly, take stock of what you might be missing. As I learned to notice my own behaviors of projecting into the future, mulling over things I couldn't control and grasping for things I didn't have yet, I realized the futility of it all.

You can teach yourself and give your life the benefit of mindfulness. It's not an ability to master overnight, but small adjustments add up. As you go, you'll discover there's real satisfaction in finishing one project before moving on to the next. It's also very respectful to give your undivided attention to the person you're talking to. Drive mindfully and you'll probably avoid many accidents. Notice when your gas tank is half full, and make a point to fill up then, rather than in the red zone when you're running late to a meeting. Take enough time to think through a week's menu and look at your pantry shelves carefully before going grocery shopping. Work from a well-prepared list when you shop to save yourself the stress of having to make another trip to the store for just one thing more. Soon you'll see a blessed contentment comes with the ability to fully enjoy the moment you're in.

<hr>

Self-Care

Wrestling with self-understanding is a human process as old as time. The psalmist said it so well: "Search me, O God, and know my heart; test me and know my anxious thoughts" (Psalm 139:23).

While you'll never know your heart as completely as God does, you can grow to understand yourself better tomorrow than you do now. I'm not talking about selfishness, self-pity, or self-indulgence, but rather an inner wisdom that you develop over time. I'm speaking of knowing yourself in the way of understanding how you work, what moves and inspires you, as well as what diminishes you or drags you down.

One of the best ways to know yourself is to learn from past or present mistakes. A good place to start is by exploring your most recent meltdown. You know what a meltdown is—when you get up in the morning and everything that can go wrong, goes wrong. The alarm didn't ring, so you get a late start. You haven't slept well in days. There's no milk in the refrigerator, and you're out of coffee. Everyone in the house seems cranky and underfoot. There's a spot on your shirt or a button missing and no time to fix it. It's raining hard and you left your car windows open last night. As you dash out of the house without an umbrella (you couldn't find one), hair getting worse by the second and makeup running, you're muttering four-letter words. You sit in the car on the verge of tears and realize the day has barely started—and it's going downhill fast. You head out of the driveway, emotionally unequipped to face the day—when what you really want to do is just go back inside and crawl under the covers, maybe permanently.

Everyone has days like these. Just the other day I witnessed a client in a meltdown, which reinforced for me the validity of knowing and caring for the self. Carol is the mother of three, a stay-at-home mom with endless household chores, which she negotiates admirably. This particular morning, however, she'd been called to help at her children's school at the last minute on one of those days where nothing goes right. She'd left baking supplies out on her kitchen counter because it was her son's birthday and she wanted to take cupcakes to his class. Of course, Carol hadn't made them yet.

When I arrived that morning I saw a tinge of anxiety in her eyes that I'd never seen before. I looked at the cupcake tins on the counter, the laundry piles on the floor, the lack of makeup on her face, and offered, "Why don't we reschedule this session for later in the week? You can use the extra hour to hop in the shower for a little self-care and get those cupcakes baked without killing yourself in the process."

Carol looked at me as if I'd just handed her a winning lottery ticket. She was able to continue her day in a different, happier frame of mind. I can bet you that she will negotiate a future day of surprises and upsets with new understanding of her own needs. I could give her the gift of an hour for herself, because I knew from personal experience an hour can make a great difference in the throes of a meltdown.

Fortunately, meltdown days do come to an end. But knowing your self helps you understand your meltdowns and how they develop—and you'll discover many are self-inflicted. In this way, knowing the self is your gift to yourself, and it has the ripple effect of gifting all the lives you touch, because no one wants to be in the path of a meltdown in progress.

As I attempted to learn from my own meltdowns, I realized there's always a pattern: Lack of sleep led to lack of energy for exercise, which led to poor food choices, which led to a bad pimple on my face. The pimple led to a feeling of defensiveness and low self-esteem, which led to a poor phone consultation with a client, which led to not getting that client. Missing out on the prospective client led to kicking myself even harder when the Visa bill came with the splurge I indulged in because I knew I had a new client starting soon. Meanwhile, something totally unrelated like a car problem or one of the dogs getting sick drops into the picture.

By reconstructing the scene of the crime, I could see clearly that I laid the foundation for the meltdown myself. Bad days were precipitated by a steady buildup of several things out of balance in my life, rather than one frustrating event. Armed with this new insight, I moved on with a renewed commitment to balance and self-care. The next challenge that comes my way—and it will come—probably won't result in a meltdown.

Every individual has unique needs for self-care in addition to some shared, common ones. Do you know yours? As you embark on knowing yourself better and integrating balance into your life, consider this checklist of basics necessary for balance. Answer the questions by writing your responses into your wellness journal or even in the margins of this page.

- How much sleep do you need to feel rested and ready to meet the day? How often do you get it?
- What's your daily water consumption? Are you getting enough or are you still dehydrated at times?
- Do you have time to sit quietly for even 10 minutes during the day, every day? How can you cultivate this?
- Do you have regular periods of solitude for thinking, writing, reading, or just puttering each day? If not, how can you provide yourself with this necessity?
- What's your passion in life? Do you get to do and enjoy it on a regular basis? Because life is short, how can you integrate what you love into your life more often?
- Who do you love? Do these people know you love them? Are they enjoying the benefit of being on your short list? How can you experience more of life's richness with them? Even a small investment of time and effort can feed a cherished relationship.
- What do you need to feel prepared each day? Do you have what you need in the refrigerator and pantry, the personal products you need—plus an extra on hand, two or more outfits that can be worn for any occasion?
- How prepared are you for financial surprises? Do you have a budget you can live with? Does your checkbook stay balanced? Do you know when you're running low on things like checks, envelopes, and stamps?
- It's good to have a plan of action for the meltdown when it comes. Do you know the name and number of a great massage therapist? Is your best friend's phone number on speed dial? Have you developed other resources of self-care that are easy to access in times of need?
- When did you last service your car? As annoying as car maintenance is, it can be less annoying than a breakdown.
- What about your own maintenance? Do you have a doctor you trust and can reach in an emergency? Do you go in for regular checkups? Do you have handy the names and numbers

of other highly recommended physicians? The best time to find a great doctor can be when you don't need one.

- **Do you have a support system?** Are family, friends, work, and church resources available to you? It helps to know who you can turn to in times of need.

It's an ongoing process to know yourself better, and change is a natural part of it. What you need in your twenties is vastly different from what you need in mid-life and beyond. The important thing is to treat your self-knowledge and self-care as a priority. Only then can you achieve a modicum of balance. There are times when it's healthier to forego an hour of exercise in order to relax in a bubble bath and paint your toenails. You can make these life-saving calls, but you have to know yourself and your needs to make them.

There is a time for everything, and a season for every activity under heaven: a time to be born and a time to die, a time to plant and a time to uproot, a time to kill and a time to heal, a time to tear down and a time to build . . .

ECCLESIASTES 3:1–3

During the year I began this book, the idea of balance went from a nice concept to something I actually experienced once in a while. Strangely, you might think at first, it began with saying wrenching goodbyes to my Uncle Huby and my Aunt Cathy. Then I greeted joyfully the arrival of two nieces—Alissa Luanne and Eileen Julianna. Then I embraced friends and relatives who came to Nashville for the occasion of my long-awaited wedding. I started a book and finished a record, worked hard but rested a lot; made two trips to Montana in the bitter cold of winter, and drove five times to my hometown in Decatur, Illinois. In July I held my oldest dog, Sax, as he breathed his last breath at age 18. But the day before Christmas Eve a tiny abandoned puppy came bouncing into my life. I turned 39 and gave up on pulling out white hairs. (Now I've learned to be affectionate toward those streaks of white and the crinkles that surround my eyes when I smile.)

So it was a year of many changes for me, but wading through so much sadness and death helped me examine my priorities. In fact, the steady stream of loss can reinforce the importance of honoring the ebb and flow so natural in life. Yet our culture, and human nature to a certain extent, seems to prefer forgetting that death is a part of life. After all, obituaries are buried in the back pages of the newspaper, and the aging process is fought with a vengeance in every magazine ad and television commercial.

I remember sitting in a social studies class in college, discussing the graying of America and plight of the elderly, thinking (at the ripe old age of 19), "Oh, that will never happen to me." The distance between teenage and twilight years was completely beyond my comprehension.

Even in my late twenties and early thirties, I was fascinated with the beautiful movie stars (especially female) whose youthful looks seemed untouched by the ravages of time. Eye jobs and other miracles of plastic surgery started to have certain appeal to me, especially as signs of the aging process started to show up in my mirror.

But in the past several years my feelings have shifted. Living in Nashville—a small town in many ways, despite its national entertainment industry—I've seen plenty of examples of cosmetic surgery and age-defying careers. On one hand I've seen up close the pathetic results of one surgery too many, and on the other the dignity and beauty of faces that have lived long and well. I've concluded: Cosmetic surgery is a tool you can use, and it's a very personal choice. But you can miss a great legacy in a person when the character lines and life history are erased from your face.

It's also a futile endeavor, anyway, to seek eternal youth. The soft, smooth face of a 20-year-old cannot be duplicated on a 45-year-old, no matter now good the surgeon; your body wasn't created to freeze in time or last forever. The reality is you're going to age over time, and one day you'll die—everyone ages, changes, and dies. There's beauty and balance in accepting this process.

129

I once read an article about Robert (*All I Really Need to Know I Learned in Kindergarten*) Fulghum, in which he talked about his antidote for bad days. He goes off to the gravesite he has chosen for himself and sits on it to reflect on life's problems. It doesn't take long for this ritual to put his day back into perspective, and he always leaves with renewed energy and enthusiasm for life.

You can cut to the bottom line in your own life without sitting on your cemetery plot or watching a loved one die. You can do it by considering the full picture of your life and the legacy you ultimately want to leave. A dear friend of mine expresses it this way, "Who will wail for me when I die? Who will say, 'You have made a difference in my life?' Who will remember my unique quirks of expression and personality?"

What qualities do you uniquely bring to the table that fill a need no one else can fill? What gifts have you been given to work with in this world? What memories have you helped create? Who will feel your passing keenly and wail for you?

I thank God that I can ask myself these questions while I still have a good portion of life to live. If I died tomorrow, I wouldn't have many regrets. That isn't something I could have said a few years ago—mainly because I was too distracted to appreciate the big picture. Today I feel the contentment of a life lived with respect for balance. It's not a perfect life without struggles, nor will it ever be. But the bad days and meltdowns just don't carry the same weight they used to. I know my strengths and weaknesses and accept them. I know I'm more than my career—that I'm a sister, daughter, wife, friend, and "mom" to six furry creatures. I feel content with the emotional investments I've made in my family and friends, and I realize a rich return from those investments daily. Perhaps the greatest gift of all has been the peace and security I've received from God now that I've time to share with him. My days end with prayer, gratitude, and silence in the presence of God.

This was the thread of grace that ran through my grandparents' lives: Each meal began with prayer, and Sunday was a day of resting and praising God. Throughout their days, Grandpa and Grandma Huber knew what really mattered, and the legacy of their traditions and time can be ours today.

The Power of Choice

Things you can do every day to impact your well-being

- **Think about the way you drive.** One dead giveaway of a life in need of balance is reckless driving. Do you regularly exceed the speed limit by more than five miles an hour? Do you weave in and out of traffic fearlessly with no regard for your safety or that of others? It's amazing how many of us behave this way. But to do this is to live on borrowed time. Think about the people who love you and depend on you the next time you flirt with death behind the steering wheel.

- **For every three times you're too busy to do something, make it a point not to be.** Everything you're in the middle of will still be there when you come back from a really great spontaneous moment. Start this practice by first noticing how often you say the words, "I'm too busy to. . . ." Consider what you're missing in life because of that. It's so human to assume you'll always have another time to do something. But those other times may never come if you don't make time.

- **Think carefully about the amount of energy a commitment will cost you in sanity and personal time.** The next time you get ready to overextend yourself with a favor, money, or work, take the time you need to mull over the effects and consequences. Learn to graciously say, "My plate is full." It becomes easier with practice, and most people will respect you for knowing your own limitations.

- **Enjoy the writings of gracious women with wisdom on how to live the good and balanced life.** Over the years I've loved the collective

131

writings of Alexandra Stoddard, whose books like *Living a Beautiful Life* and *Daring to be Yourself* give countless ways on how to create sanctuary in your home—both realistically and affordably. Stoddard's sense of style and love for life come through every page. Also, if you've not yet read Anne Morrow Lindberg's *Gift from the Sea,* get a copy to read today. It's remarkable that this book, first published some 50 years ago, still has so much to say about the balancing act women have performed throughout the ages—and it's incredibly insightful for our challenging times.

- **Don't let your exercise routine become one of those things that keeps you too busy to do things with people you love.** Yes, exercise is important to health, but never more important than the other components of wellness, and when it's out of balance it's downright unhealthy.

Six

Emotional Health

Confront the dark parts of yourself,
and work to banish them
with illumination and forgiveness.
Your willingness to wrestle
with your demons will cause
your angels to sing.

ANGUS WILSON

A tall, slender woman with striking features and a winning smile walks into the aerobics room of a fitness club to prepare for a low-impact workout class. Outgoing and confident, she greets participants and cues her music. She looks healthy, without an ounce of fat on her body, which is set off perfectly by the leotard she wears. She teaches with energy and enthusiasm and makes herself available after class for questions and feedback.

Every aspect of her performance exudes professionalism, her love for people, and her high standards for her work. Many of her students consider her to be multi-talented and tell her they want to be like her some day.

What they don't know, though, is how this woman struggles with perfectionism, dissatisfaction with her life, and deep-rooted emotional pain. In fact, if they followed her home from work, they'd quickly cease wanting to be like her.

After she's straightened the aerobics room, she's tired—more than she ever lets on to a class, or anyone else for that matter. She heads home, lets herself into her apartment, and checks for messages on the answering machine. There are a few calls, but none for performances that weekend, so she worries that her musical career isn't moving ahead. The aerobics classes are just part-time, you see. She really wants a record deal, to be a star, and if she can just realize that dream, she'll have the life she's always wanted, the money she needs, and the positive reinforcement she craves to feel good about herself.

For now there's just this tiny apartment, a phone that doesn't ring, and bills that get more overwhelming each month. Since it's early evening, she jumps into the shower to clean off the sweat from her workout with the class. She's close to starting her menstrual cycle and feels bloated, a little puffy through the abdomen and hips, so she decides to get on the scale, just to see what she weighs. The number is about three pounds over her comfort zone.

The tiredness, loneliness, lack of the work she wants, and slight weight gain combine to send her into a downward spiral. She showers and has dinner, but the healthy meal she prepares can't satisfy her need for comfort. So she continues to eat: a full carton of ice cream, a package of cookies, granola from a just-opened box—a big bowl of it smothered in half-and-half.

One hour later she's through eating. That is, after consuming French toast covered with maple syrup and the rest of the box of granola. She's eaten and eaten until her stomach is distended like a pregnant woman's and beads of sweat cover her brow. Her aerobics class wouldn't recognize her now. Miserable and hating herself, she goes to the bathroom to repeat a familiar ritual, one that's dogged her for years. She leans over the sink, turns on the water, tickles the back of her throat with her finger, and throws up. It takes her 15 minutes to undo the eating of the past two hours.

Wearily, she gets back into the shower for a symbolic cleansing, and cries as the water washes over her battered body and mouth. Then she falls into bed, exhausted. *Maybe that was it,* she thinks as she drifts off to sleep. *Maybe this was the last time.* She vows to herself, *I'll do better tomorrow. I'll start over again tomorrow.*

This woman could be you or someone you know. Twenty-five percent of young American women, from their teenage years on, struggle with an eating disorder—a statistic that's steadily increased over the last few decades. But I'm familiar with this woman because more than 15 years ago she was me. I was on my way to recovery from a struggle with the bulimia that had plagued me intermittently since my early twenties. But I wasn't there yet.

This is a difficult topic to broach, because most of us would like to think messy terms like "bulimia," alcoholism," and "sexual abuse" only affect other people. Yet the cycles of addiction and codependence

135

are pervasive in our culture; during your lifetime you'll know and love someone who is struggling with emotional pain.

However, striving for wellness without addressing emotional health is an exercise in futility. Unresolved emotional pain will eventually take its toll on the body, regardless of how much that body is exercised or how perfectly it's fed. One might achieve temporary weight loss while remaining emotionally unhealthy, but it will be short-lived, because no diet, food plan, amount of exercise, or self-discipline will ever counteract the weight gain that comes from an obsession with food.

I encourage you to open yourself to the possibility that emotional healing is a valid process.

Every form of addiction is bad, . . . whether the narcotic be
alcohol or morphine or idealism.

CARL GUSTAV JUNG

Sandy, a single, 37-year-old woman who works at a day-care center, has experienced this. She enjoys her work and has a special gift with children. In fact, she'd like to have a family of her own someday, but she's never had a serious relationship with a man that could lead to marriage. She's too busy and distracted with her addiction to compulsive eating and dieting. The 30 extra pounds she wears on her body provide an armor of protection against intimacy, and this stems from an incident of sexual abuse during childhood, which she refuses to dwell upon. "That's all in the past," she figures. She blames herself. *It was probably my fault anyway,* she thinks, a memory that instills shame. She doesn't want to revisit that memory. She just wants to lose those 30 stubborn pounds and get on with her life.

She's tried every diet, every exercise program, and still she can't stabilize her weight. Deep in her heart she knows she is powerless over her need to eat for reasons other than hunger, but she can't just admit she needs professional help. She chalks her weight gain up to a lack of self-control and stays in denial. It might not be a perfect life, but it's a familiar one—and at times oddly comforting.

Many times I've worked with other clients fighting the same battle. At some point I ask them to keep a food diary or take responsibility for an extra session of cardiovascular exercise between our workouts. For one reason or another they just cannot follow through on these assignments. Their resistance to keeping food intake records or fitting a 20-minute walk into their schedule reveals a need to stay right where they are in life.

People who routinely overeat for reasons other than hunger can be extraordinarily organized in other parts of their lives. But they can't seem to confront the real reason for their overeating or neglect to exercise. They're still in denial over the issues that paralyze them, and they're more comfortable taking the blame for lack of self-control than admitting they're addicted to food.

I can encourage them to explore the reasons they eat and in time get to a peaceful place with food, but it won't have any effect. I can share the example of my own recovery from food addiction and the hope I feel for anyone in that struggle. But if clients aren't ready, they remain unfazed by any words. Denial keeps them right where they are, trapped in their addictions, thinking that recovery is for other people and therapy would never work for them.

The word "addiction" covers a lot of territory and is slippery to define. It can conjure up images of a drunk passed out on the street, or the needle-scarred arm of a heroin addict, or maybe a scene from *The Days of Wine and Roses*. But there are many forms of addiction and countless ways to be addicted. Researchers have documented chemical dependency on alcohol, drugs, and nicotine over the years and have widely acknowledged these substances are really addictive agents. But the spectrum of addictions in our society is much broader than the abuse of alcohol, drugs, and cigarettes. Food, sex, love, money, shopping, work, rage, exercise, success, power, fame, control, relationships, and even religion can pull you into an addiction that disrupts your life as much as any chemical dependence.

Denial can work hand-in-hand with an addiction to keep you in a holding pattern. After all, even though an addiction can't ultimately satisfy or fulfill you, it can temporarily distract you from deep-rooted pain and the issues causing it. So most people have a vested interest to remain in the holding pattern of addiction, especially when the thing they're addicted to has the illusion of being virtuous or is even socially acceptable.

Many young women fall into this trap—women like Susie, a bright, straight-A honors student at a prestigious university. Attractive and healthy-looking, Susie seems to excel at everything she does. She exercises like clockwork every day. Her routine includes a 6:00 A.M. aerobics class, a workout with weights at the gym during lunch, and a five-mile run after classes each evening. But she's obsessed with her workouts and gets distracted and upset when something prevents her from exercising on schedule.

For Susie, exercise is like a drug. She'll choose it over other activities, friendships, and even at the risk of her own well-being. She'll wrap a painful knee or ankle and run on an injury rather than take off time to rest and heal. The longer she remains influenced by this socially acceptable addiction, the more it will disrupt her life and damage her body. It will keep her from enjoying a balanced life and get in the way of having relationships. Despite these negatives, exercise represents a means of control that she's terrified to give up.

Early in my fitness career, when Vanderbilt University was in session and coeds stormed the aerobics studio where I worked, I saw a lot of women like Susie. Exercise addiction among college students is common and frequently mistaken for healthy behavior. Only the behavior of the girls who came to my 4:15 P.M. aerobics class was anything but healthy. Their locker room conversations were chilling to overhear. One coed would squeeze nonexistent fat on her hips and make disparaging remarks about her body. Another would get on the scale, then step down, and declare she wasn't going to eat again until she'd lost five pounds.

I witnessed these scenes countless times before and after classes, and it filled me with sadness. These were energetic twenty-somethings funneling their youth and vitality into an obsession with weight and exercise. I knew what they were going through and how much of life they were missing, trapped in their addictions. The fact that our culture encourages this only made the situation all the more pitiable. And yet addiction and denial don't recognize socioeconomic boundaries nor discriminate. Walk into any home, church, or workplace—wealthy, cultured, or not—and you'll see signs of the addictive process. I saw amazing examples while working the society-gig circuit in Nashville.

One of the hosts I regularly entertained with my music was routinely inebriated before his dinner parties even began. His drinking started with wine at lunch, followed by cocktails at 5:00 P.M. He was a wealthy, sophisticated, and successful businessman with well-developed interests in art, music, and gourmet food—and the resources to enjoy them. But I never played a party for him that he wasn't falling-down drunk by the end of the night.

The thing that used to amaze me about this wealthy client was that he was surrounded by people who liked him but seemed content to let him live out his disease. He had all the resources necessary to check into the best treatment center in the country. The fact that neither his friends nor family would intervene to help amazes me to this day.

When I struggled with my eating disorder I also went through a long period of denial by thinking: *If my life just went the way I envision, if I just weighed the right amount, I would be happy, and this food stuff would go away.* I've watched other strugglers do this too. They'll resist the therapeutic process and cling to the false belief that their weight problems or other issues could be solved by a new approach, a fresh start, more money, or heightened prayer. There's great resistance to getting help in our culture. But addiction can fell the most capable and intelligent of people. The walking wounded are everywhere, flailing through life without seeking help, inflicting the pain of their codependence on others, especially those they love.

<hr />

Codependence provides us all . . . with a clearer and expanded way of describing the dynamic that underlies most neuroses, addictions and other disorders. It is the human condition.

CHARLES L. WHITFIELD, M.D., FROM
CO-DEPENDENCE, HEALING THE HUMAN CONDITION

One hundred million Americans across two concurrent generations suffer problems of what's been called the mother of all addictions—codependency, according to authors Robert Hemfelt, Frank Minirth, and Paul Meier in their book *Love Is a Choice*. In fact, the authors write, "Codependency is an epidemic." No one is immune; codependency affects each of us in today's world in one way or another, taking a huge toll on health, family, and the fabric of society.

You can see codependence upon not just drugs and alcohol, but compulsive exercise and eating, unhealthy relationships, and all sorts of things. You see it with the routine abuse of money and power in politics and government, or the compulsive spending that racks up huge credit card debts, and in unreasonable displays of anger or acts of violence that make the six o'clock news every night—and these are just a few signs of this disease witnessed every day.

The term "codependence" first gained acceptance in the psycho-therapy community during the 1970s. But the quest for recognizing and treating the emotional dysfunction goes back another one hundred years or so—to the time of Freud, Jung, and other pioneers of research into the human psyche. At first the term referred to the condition of the caretaker or enabler of a person suffering from alcoholism or drug dependency. Since the late 1980s, however, almost every addiction and compulsive behavior can be linked to this underlying disease.

So what is codependence exactly? The word is broadly defined. It can be described as an inherited or acquired emotional illness, which begins in childhood and gets reinforced along life's path. But one of the best definitions I've heard is this: "Codependence is a flawed belief that by using or controlling substances, situations, and people outside ourselves we can change the way we feel on the inside."

This perception of life is learned very early, usually by the age of six, and gathers momentum as a person grows into adulthood. It's even possible to live a lifetime under the influence of codependence, but it's a sad waste, because living with codependence is like walking through life wearing eyeglasses made out of bottle glass. You see just enough to get around, but you're missing the real shape, color, and clarity of life and all its beauty.

Psychologists and therapists have been working with people in recovery from codependence for nearly thirty years. Books like *Codependent No More* by Melody Beattie, the collective writings of John Bradshaw, and *Love Is a Choice* are just a few of the classic resources available to help explain and demystify this pervasive disease.

But if you want to live a whole, unfettered life, you must do more than read about codependence. You must acknowledge the role it plays in your personal history and gain some understanding of the disease. My contribution isn't that of a therapist or psychologist, but as a member of the walking wounded who, by God's infinite mercy, got better.

Those who know something is amiss in their lives sometimes ask me, as a Christian, "Don't you believe that God can heal your pain if you have faith and pray for help?"

I give God complete credit for saving my life. I believe he sent the people, money, therapists, and support systems I needed to start and continue down the path to healing. Miraculous, emotional healing can occur, but answers to our prayers don't usually manifest themselves without our participation. Very few of us, for instance, would expect to be spontaneously healed of a broken bone just by praying.

There are countless ways to avoid this process and many excuses: "Oh, it costs too much. . . ." "Our marriage isn't so bad; look at everyone else's. . . ." "How could going to therapy possibly help me control my weight? . . ." "No one in our family has ever had to get help; why should I be the first one?"

Other people resist the therapeutic path because they think codependence denotes a shortcoming or weakness in the individual. People don't want to include themselves in the category of recovering codependent, because they think it labels them as a loser. This is understandable.

Unfortunately codependence, like anything else, has received its share of bad press. I'll never forget a well-known television personality's introduction of a millionaire who owned a giant corporation. The interview followed a segment on codependence, and the first words out of this personality's mouth were, "You can call the subject of our next feature many things, but one thing's for sure—he's not codependent."

I was appalled. That simple comment proved to me that this correspondent had no understanding of codependence, because the subject of her interview was a well-known workaholic and control addict—both classic signs of codependence! Also wealth and fame don't rule out codependence; if anything they attract it. So why is it that codependence is something expected only to be in the life of a loser?

Think about it. Many people whom we laud and admire are, or at some time have been, in the grips of addiction and codependence: artists, musicians, actors, great writers past and present, statesmen, presidents and world leaders, movie and television stars, comedians, Fortune 500 executives, the ranks of the socially elite, country, rock, and pop personalities.

Now think of people closer to home, people you might know. The lady at church who does everything for everyone else at the expense of her own health. The mother who drives her children to countless lessons and activities, keeps her house spotless, wears all the right clothes, and says all the right things, but has a nervous breakdown. The charming, handsome, and financially successful man who's married several times but never finds peace in his relationships.

As Charles L. Whitfield has observed, codependence is "the human condition."

In the midst of these bleak observations on humanity, it's easy to feel a degree of futility or lack of hope. But acknowledging that things are the way they are opens the door to changing them. Back in 1935 with the founding of Alcoholics Anonymous and the Twelve-Step Program, a new era of human thought was born. The Twelve Steps, based on biblical thought, teach us to turn the control of our lives back over to God and commit to a process of self-examination.

In taking the therapeutic path, you can admit it's not enough to just live your life but to examine it. That examination process helps disarm the power of addiction and denial. It encourages a complete surrender to God and an ongoing personal and moral inventory. The beneficial process of self-examination will lead to a therapeutic path if it's supposed to—and this path begins with understanding the impact of your childhood experiences on determining the course of your life. Marsha's story illustrates this perfectly.

The Scars
of Childhood

Marsha is a capable and outgoing woman in her late thirties, married, with two children. Her husband has a high-paying job in the insurance business. Neighbors and friends at church admire this family. But Marsha has a secret no one suspects. Her likeable, easygoing husband routinely rages at her with explosive anger. She lives in constant fear of his next physical assault.

Marsha's learned how to hide the signs of her abuse with cleverly arranged clothes, makeup, and hair, and she fools even her closest friends with her effusive good nature. But in an unguarded moment, when she's tired or worried about her children, she has a bruised look about her. It's the same look her mother wore for most of her life.

You see, Marsha learned very early not to tell about the undercurrents at home. As a child she'd witnessed the violent behavior of her father, a church deacon, as he struck and berated her mother on a regular basis. Like many children who observe violence in the family, Marsha assumed the role of caretaker and rescuer early on: She tried to diffuse and distract her father's anger, rescue her mother, and master looking good on the outside to preserve the family image of unreproachable perfection.

Marsha survived her childhood physically but entered adulthood and her own marriage with a twisted perception of life. As a codependent she displays the characteristics of a care-aholic, a perfectionist, and a control addict. Her childhood has taught her to elevate the needs of others above her own and take the blame and responsibility for the pain and anger of her husband. Marsha has no reference point for a healthy relationship between adults or between a parent and a child. All she knows is the dysfunction of her parents' home and now her own.

Perhaps someday Marsha will break through to the realization that she can't fix or control her husband's anger. Or perhaps a friend or family member will intervene to remove Marsha from her role as a

143

human punching bag. One thing's for sure: If she doesn't get help, her children will be destined for the same cycle of pain and abuse, because codependence doesn't go away with time. As Carl Jung observed, it only gets stronger. "Nothing," he said, "has a stronger influence psychologically on their environment and especially on their children than the unlived life of the parent."

In the beginning of my therapeutic process, I can remember being skeptical about my childhood experiences having anything to do with the current mess in my life. I couldn't see any obvious sign that I'd lived through anything but the most normal, uneventful experiences: My parents never fought, no one came home drunk, there was no violence, no broken home. "Besides, how could something that happened thirty years ago have any bearing on my present situation?" I asked.

This is a natural reaction at the outset of the recovery process. Many people feel reluctant to dishonor or hurt their families when they start therapy. They'll say things like, "Well, I know my father was cruel and abusive—but what good does it do to complain about that or blame him for the way my life is today?"

If all you ever experienced from the moment of birth was the pure, unconditional love of God, you wouldn't know codependency, dysfunction, or addiction. After all, when you're born you're equipped with everything you need to be a healthy, whole, authentic individual. But you're born of human parents, and at birth you immediately begin to gather countless signals and messages about life from them and others. Like a sponge, you absorb and internalize every sensation, feeling, and experience; by the time you start school, you've already learned your foundational beliefs and skills for navigating life.

You can see how learned skills play out in the life of one boy who grows up in a family with a mother, father, and three younger sisters. The boy's father is a needy man with low self-esteem, who married the boy's mother after breaking her heart and later reconciling. The mother never resolved the pain and anger from her own youth, nor entirely recovered from the rocky start to her marriage.

So the young boy learns very early in life that he must support and esteem his father and ease the pain and anger in his mother. He also learns to be the strong steady pillar in the family for his three younger sisters. By the time he's eight, he's completely abandoned himself to be a caretaker and protector. He's learned that the world is not a safe place and he can depend on no one. He's learned to ignore his own needs and feelings in lieu of the needs and feelings of others. He's got a heightened sense of control and responsibility and believes he can change the world around him with his caretaking: He can encourage his father and diffuse his father's selfish nature. He can make his mother feel better. He can protect his sisters from any harm that comes their way.

Do you see the big problem here? Young boys or girls are not supposed to shoulder the emotional responsibility of keeping the family unit happy. This young boy should be looking to his father for support and self-esteem, not the other way around. He deserves to have a mother who takes care of her own anger and pain. He needs siblings who take turns supporting each other and helping out in the family unit. But this boy doesn't experience those healthy things. He continues to grow, with a negative feeling about life (it's hard and unfair) and becomes a master of repressing his own feelings of pain.

By the time he's a teenager, his coping mechanisms are well in place. He's completely cut off from his authentic self, which never had a chance to develop, and operates from the primary scenario of his childhood. When his mother dies suddenly in an auto accident, the expectations he has for life are cemented: Bad things happen, life is random and unfair, and it is better not to feel than to suffer from the pain. At the funeral he is barely able to grieve. But it is no surprise, because this boy learned to stop feeling a long time ago.

The boy becomes a young man and eventually marries a vivacious and capable woman. Together they have three children, all girls, whom they raise in a solid Christian home. Here's where the trickle-down effect of codependence rears its ugly head. None of the girls ever experiences obvious signs of abuse or addiction in their family home. But as young children, they observe their father's shutdown, repressed nature and their mother's whirlwind of caretaking as she frantically tries to make up for his lack of emotion. Being the acutely attuned creatures that children are, they innately understand that Dad is depressed and that it's their job to somehow make him feel better. Their codependence takes hold early, and it's an even stronger version than their father knew. Later in their lives, the disease plays itself out in various forms of depression, love hunger, broken marriages, and alcohol addiction. Unless they're able to resolve this multigenerational pain, they'll in turn pass it onto their own children, with concentrated strength.

No parent has ever received ideal parenting or given perfect love to his or her own children. We've all been wounded in some way and more often than not by parents trying to do their very best. Revisiting the wounds of childhood is not an exercise in parent bashing. It's more an exercise in understanding how you or I received the wounds we did, and it's about healing those wounds in order to live as whole, healthy adults.

<hr />

The life which is unexamined is not worth living.

PLATO

I can remember the very day my personal recovery from codependence and addiction began. It was sunny and breezy in Nashville, and I was sitting on the back stairway exit of the aerobics studio between teaching a 4:15 and 5:15 class. The studio manager sat with me. She'd been recently interviewed on local television about her personal recovery from an eating disorder, and I told her—the first person ever—that I knew what she'd been through, that I too suffered from an eating problem. In one conversation that lasted less than fifteen minutes, I moved forward a light year in my healing. I'd broken the silence about my own disease and started a dialogue about my eating disorder with someone I could trust and who could be part of my support system. It would be another year before I started therapy, but my process of recovery had begun.

The therapeutic process is as unique to you as a thumbprint. Sometimes it begins with a sudden realization that life shouldn't be this hard, and you desire to experience life differently, whatever it takes.

Sometimes a core issue will suddenly explode, sending you crawling into therapy for immediate attention. My path had elements of both.

With my friend's help and support I started and maintained abstinence from bingeing and purging. I began exploring books on recovery and treating myself with a little more care. To encourage myself I pinned positive affirmations about love, abundance, and self-esteem all over the walls of my apartment. My network of friends grew to include people who were in therapy and were making positive changes in their lives, which I witnessed with respect. But I'd only scratched the surface of my addictive nature and emotional pain. I had released some steam from the pressure cooker inside, and God had provided me with resources and a sense of safety, but the pressure was still building and the pain was not resolved.

The pressure cooker finally exploded on a summer weekend fifteen years ago. A turbulent relationship I'd been involved in for a few years came to an abrupt, unpleasant end. I lay on the floor of my apartment and wailed like a wounded animal. I was incapable of functioning. For weeks my eyes were red-rimmed and swollen, and I couldn't do anything without bursting into tears. The second stage of my therapeutic process had begun.

Adversity stripped away denial, leaving me with a new willingness to search my soul. As the American poet Theodore Roethke said, "In a dark time, the eye begins to see."

Still, as willing as I now was to walk through whatever I had to, I resisted the exploration of my childhood. I labored under the delusion that my pain was related only to the breakup of this relationship.

During one session, as the therapist tried to draw out deeper issues, I blurted, "I just don't think I can survive if my boyfriend never comes back to me."

The therapist said matter of factly, "Oh, you just want to talk about your boyfriend, well, that's OK."

It was then that I realized the pain of the breakup was only a symptom of something deeper, much bigger. As hard as it was to focus my attention on those core issues, I understood the necessity of it. Slowly, I confronted the layers of pain. After a while I was able to understand the reasons I was the way I was.

147

Therapy is like going back to college and majoring in the self. For a recovering codependent it is a real exercise in looking inside for truth and meaning instead of whirling around, constantly trying to manipulate people and situations to make things feel better. I learned that I had depended on things like work, love relationships, and control—as well as food—to provide relief and distraction from my pain. The hurt of the breakup was a symptom of my control addiction. Surrendering control was very hard, because it had been my main source of medication for many years. I was always the one who broke things off. Having my boyfriend decide for both of us that the relationship was over was terrible.

Control is a process addiction, not a substance-related addiction, but the withdrawal from it is just as debilitating. I had been obsessed with getting this boyfriend back. Because I was in therapy, I knew I had to abstain from that behavior, but I still felt compelled to talk about him, hear about him, fantasize about seeing him again—just like a recovering alcoholic craving a drink.

A few close friends talked me off what felt like being on the edge of the cliff several times a day. They helped save my life with their patience and empathy. We can laugh about it now, and we refer to it as "that terrible summer." Giving up control was a big step, but recognizing it and understanding what drove it facilitated my recovery.

Navigating a personal relationship under the influence of codependence is like trying to get close to someone while draped head-to-toe in a wool blanket. The cloak of the disease shades the way we deal with people and how they deal with us. It can also affect our health. Insomnia, chronic pain, migraine headaches, digestive problems, fatigue, and depression are commonly driven by emotional issues.

Emotional pain finds refuge in the cells of the body when it cannot be released and expressed. Anyone who grew up in a family environment that didn't encourage the healthy release of anger, sadness, and joy learned to hold feelings inside. But emotions and feelings need to move through the body, as naturally as breathing in air and breathing it out.

There are healthy and appropriate ways to express every emotion we experience, but most of us don't learn how to do this while growing up.

148

Instead we learn how to shut down and disassociate ourselves from those feelings—a classic symptom of codependence. Over years and years of shutting down and emotionally disappearing, the body will finally rebel. If the disease cannot get our attention by messing up our lives enough to demand a change, then sometimes it will show up as a physical symptom. Codependence has a life of its own and is self-protective, but it will eventually create enough discomfort to demand healing.

Ultimately the healing process clears out the internal space that was once cluttered up by the disease. It's not unlike draining a festering wound, then disinfecting it, and giving it air to heal.

After wading through some substantial issues, I started to feel physically better. My back stopped going out, my skin cleared up, my sleep improved, and I didn't feel so bone-tired all the time. The therapeutic process gave me the ability to negotiate a whole new way of life.

Today I recognize my obsessive-compulsive tendencies more easily. I can give a name and expression to the feelings I used to medicate with food and control. It's not that the hurt places or dark parts of me ever go away. I just have a healthier, whole person with which to encompass them.

When I first started counseling, a dear friend who sponsored some of it said to me many times, "Ruth, I'm so glad you're giving yourself this gift." I didn't understand that at first, because it felt as if she was giving me the gift.

Now I understand perfectly. The process of recovery is a gift that only you can give yourself.

Let's not get into paralysis through analysis. Let's leave some space for God to walk through the room.
QUINCY JONES

When I consider my life and the way I lived it before I started my healing process, I'm amazed I got to this point in one piece. The person I used to be seems like a very bad dream. God intervened many times to keep me from self-destruction, I'm convinced. Most people who get to the other side of the healing path feel the same way. The world just feels like a different place on the other side.

A friend once described the exploration and rooting out process as "walking through a cleansing fire." I would say this is a pretty accurate description of recovery from addiction and codependence. When the journey starts it can also feel a lot like lifting the lid off of our personal Pandora's Box—once it's started, there's no turning back. Awareness leads to exploration, and the rollercoaster ride begins. But it's not a ride you take alone, because God is with you and me through all the peaks and valleys. He wants us to find healing, and ultimately, his peace.

I discovered firsthand that there's no way to predict how long the process will take or what all will be involved. Just three weeks into therapy I asked, "How long is this going to take?"

"Ruth," my therapist said, "some people are in therapy for six years or more." Recovery, it was explained, is ongoing and usually spans several years.

Aghast at that notion, I determined then and there to get through my therapy in three months. Well, two years of individual counseling, one year of group therapy, and several years of couple counseling (interspersed throughout) gave me a new humility about the path to wholeness.

Long stretches on this path feel awful. You do get to the other side, but it can be three steps forward and two steps back over much of the journey. Yet every step of the way gleans new understanding and develops new tools for immediate use. You realize every stumble and setback is worthwhile, because this path leads directly to God.

You'll never arrive at a perfect destination. Your challenges and problems won't end. What will change is your perception of the things that happen to you, your abilities to negotiate them, and your behavior throughout. The things that used to make your life unmanageable no longer have the same pull. The examination of your life doesn't end, but it becomes less time consuming. The walk is less of the world and more with God. Surrender to his wisdom and his control is easier, quicker. The spiritual path becomes a more natural choice.

This beautiful and famous prayer by Protestant theologian Reinhold Niebuhr—a prayer known for years in the recovery movement as the Serenity Prayer—tells you everything you need to know about recovery from codependence: "God, grant us the serenity to accept the things we cannot change, the courage to change the things we can and the wisdom to know the difference." I like to paraphrase it this way: "God, I cannot live for even one day without your grace. I surrender my life and my shortcomings to you. . . . Grant me the serenity to accept the things I have no control over—other people, their thoughts, feelings, and actions. Grant me the courage to change the only things I can ever change—my perceptions, my behavior, myself. Grant me the wisdom each day to know the difference between this truth and the pull of my human nature."

If you're on the therapeutic journey, you have my prayers and admiration. If you've not yet found the way, I wish for you, in your own time, the beautiful, freeing experience of self-examination. "We shall never cease from exploration," the poet T. S. Eliot gently reminds, "and the end of all our exploring will be to arrive where we started and know the place for the first time."

The Power of Choice
Things you can do every day to impact your well-being

The emotional healing process is extremely personal, and everyone who embarks on it finds their own way. These ideas can open doors to healing and self-examination.

- **Start a journal to explore and express feelings** about where your life is today and what experiences had the greatest impact on you in the past. Keep this journal in a safe, private place so you can express yourself without fear or inhibition. Writing down your thoughts, feelings, and insights is extremely helpful in the process of self-examination.

- **Be aware of how much time you have alone to be still.** Emotional healing generally cannot happen in the midst of chaotic, busy schedules, and staying overly busy is one of the ways many people use to avoid dealing with their issues. Carve out time for long, leisurely walks outdoors, days you can turn off the phone and be a hermit, and retreat into your safest environment to rest and pamper yourself. Rent your favorite movies and eat popcorn. Enjoy a luxurious bubble bath. By treating yourself with gentleness and care, your body and mind will begin to believe that healing is an option.

- **Write a no-holds barred letter to release pent-up feelings of pain and frustration,** negative emotions that can take a toll on the body. Is there someone in your life that you'd like to tell a few things, but can't find a safe or appropriate way to do this? Get what you need off your chest and into words, onto paper, then keep that letter in a safe place or burn it. This can also be a way to find closure with someone in your life who has died, with whom you have unfinished business.

- **Think of what you might have lost as a child and what activities could symbolically replace that**—especially since codependence tends to force children into adult roles at an early age. Part of the recovery process includes healing and restoring parts of your lost childhood. Playing with coloring books, paint sets, clay, scrapbooks, and other kinds of art are a natural place to start.

- **Set boundaries as a big step toward experiencing an emotionally healthy life.** By boundaries I mean, practice the ability to say "no" when you mean "no," instead of automatically saying "yes" to meet another person's needs. You must care of yourself if you want to have something healthy and genuine to offer others; by setting boundaries you honor your own limitations and avoid getting overextended and frustrated.

- **Learn to ask for what you need**—another big step toward emotional health. There's nothing wrong with asking for a favor or some assistance from someone you trust. It took me forever to start exercising this skill, but what a difference it makes. We all take turns helping, asking, leaning, supporting, giving, and taking in this life. Be willing to make yourself vulnerable and you'll discover it's a wonderful way to discover that life doesn't have to be so solitary and hard.

Seven

Self-Responsibility

*Responsible persons are mature
people who have taken charge
of themselves and their conduct,
who own their actions and own up
to them—who answer for them.*

WILLIAM J. BENNETT IN *THE BOOK OF VIRTUES*

In *The Book of Virtues*, a collection of classic moral literature, William J. Bennett offers examples of and commentary on fundamental character traits like self-discipline, compassion, responsibility, courage, honesty, loyalty, and other virtues that most people share a respect for. Each story, poem, and essay in this wonderful book reflects the triumph of the human spirit as it transcends the shortcomings of human nature. Regarding the virtue of responsibility, Bennett states, "In the end, we are answerable for the kinds of persons we have made of ourselves."

These words ring true as a prerequisite for wellness—a sense of self-responsibility for one's health. In fact, self-responsibility is crucial to health and happiness. Like any virtue, self-responsibility can be embraced as a way of life or ignored. By embracing it you acknowledge that your choices have ramifications and your actions impact your life in a direct, profound way. Choosing to be self-responsible makes a statement about how you perceive your place in the world. It's reflected in the way you treat yourself and respond to challenges.

Note how the elements of wellness weave in and out of each other, interacting and connecting to create health. Motivation acts as a springboard for action and an ingredient of staying power for lifestyle change. Exercise, food, and water are intricately connected to weight control, energy, and physical stamina. Balance is necessary to honor the body's need for rest and the human need for sanity and serenity. Emotional stability and health provide the ability to navigate life's great challenges, unfettered by addiction and dysfunction.

Self-responsibility is the backbone in the pursuit of wellness: It's a sign of maturity and healthy self-esteem, and it's the character trait that separates doers from dreamers, victors from victims, and the proactive from the reactive. When you make self-responsibility a way of life, empowerment and freedom result.

We have a tradition in my family: We wash our own laundry, we raise our own children, and we clean up our own dirt.

ALICE SILVERMAN

When Grandpa and Grandma Huber married in 1913, they innately understood the principle of self-responsibility. They knew, for instance, that they could depend only on their own diligence and hard work to put food on the table. My grandpa knew that if a field was to be planted or a fence to be fixed, he would have to do it himself. My grandma knew that if the abundance of a good harvest was to be realized, she would have to can and preserve that food in a timely manner. This sense of self-responsibility was reflected in the way they lived and the way they raised their children. My grandparents knew they would receive from life only that which they put into it, and they never shirked from making the appropriate investments.

Today's world is different. Self-reliance is not as crucial for survival as in my grandparents' time, nor is it emulated consistently in our culture. But as a principle, self-responsibility has merit and timelessness. Like any other virtue or positive characteristic, self-responsibility has to be understood and learned. Some people learn it earlier in life, while others never learn it at all. The extent to which you exercise this virtue is evident in the way you approach your work, daily activities, and personal conduct. Over the span of a lifetime it's also reflected by the way you treat your body and your health.

Consider what self-responsibility means in the most general sense. When you're young, usually by kindergarten, you learn there are certain things in life you're accountable for, basic skills of self-responsibility like making your bed, picking up your room, and using good manners. You learn to say "please" when you ask for something and "thank you" when you receive it. You begin to understand that there

157

are consequences to your actions and many things in life you have to answer for.

Later you learn self-responsibility in more specific ways. If homework is assigned in class, you must complete it and turn it in on time. If you're given chores to do around the house, or babysitting jobs, you must follow through with the appropriate efforts or face the consequences. You learn that certain behaviors like lying, cheating, and stealing are unacceptable and can have dire effects on your life—and others'. By the time you reach adulthood, you understand that your choices can bring you pleasure or pain, further your career or destroy it, help keep your family together or contribute to breaking it apart. You learn that in many ways you can live or die by your own hand.

———◦◦◦———

No man is in true health who cannot stand in the free air of heaven,
with his feet on God's free turf, and thank his Creator
for the simple luxury of physical existence.
T. W. HIGGINSON

Self-responsibility is every bit as applicable to your health and well-being as it is to the way you conduct your professional and personal life. Like anything else you enjoy in the day-to-day—the relationships dear to you, home you live in, car you drive—your health and well-being require attention and care. After all you're born with a magnificent body (made in the image of God), given the priceless gift from him of a life to live, and the choice to make the best or worst of it.

Of course it's easy to take your body for granted because of all it does for you. But the fact is, the choices you make every day affect your health, either taking you in the direction of long life or the direction of premature death.

For that reason it's good to revisit two important choices explored earlier in this book: being physically active and eating low on the food chain. Dr. Kenneth Cooper acknowledges this when he says, "If I were to tell you that we have developed this new pill and you can take one tablet a day and reduce death from heart attacks, strokes, diabetes, and cancer by 55 percent, and increase your life span by two and a half years, we could not manufacture enough pills."

That magic pill doesn't exist, of course. But Dr. Cooper's talking about the results that can be achieved by walking two miles in thirty minutes, three times a week.

The same observation about the power of choice can be made about practicing reasonable nutrition. You're the final arbiter of what gets from the supermarket, refrigerator, or restaurant, and onto your plate. Why not honor the good lifestyle choices that most of the time can keep you out of the doctor's office and fully in the functional and productive life God wants for you? This is the first step toward self-responsibility, after all: understanding how your lifestyle choices have consequences—and how to make good ones.

Implementing the power of choice means more than how much you exercise or eat, however. Every day you make decision in other areas of life that impact your physical, emotional, and spiritual well-being.

Choose to Be Tobacco Free

If you smoke or use tobacco products, this is where your path to wellness begins. Well-documented evidence links both smoking and tobacco use to greater risk of cancer and heart disease. Having worked in the Vanderbilt Cancer Clinic Volunteer Program at times, I've seen firsthand the ravaging results of tobacco use. Now whenever I see someone smoking I feel an urge to get down on my knees and beg them to quit. I've never actually done this, but I've longed to say, "You are too precious in God's sight to destroy yourself with tobacco."

Granted, quitting isn't easy. Nicotine is so powerfully addictive that 52 million Americans are hooked on it. But know that any efforts made toward wellness—like exercising or eating well—are gutted by smoking. Is there any reason then for a self-responsible adult to smoke at all or to not make it a priority to quit?

Fortunately, there are many resources for help (like The American Heart Association and The American Cancer Society), and a lot of them are free. This is good news for anyone with a desire to live the good life.

Use Alcohol in Moderation, If at All

Substance abuse is such an insidious problem in this country, you're well advised to take a serious look—using caution and respect—at the way you use alcoholic beverages. A glass of good wine with dinner is one of life's great pleasures, but like any mood-altering substance, it has an addictive pull. If you choose to drink, be mindful of how much, how often, and why. Look at your family history for signs of alcohol abuse or other health disorders that might contraindicate your own use of it. Be aware that although there's evidence wine may be beneficial to health, there's no such evidence regarding hard liquor. Consider limiting yourself to no more than five drinks a week and practicing regular periods of abstinence from alcoholic beverages in general.

Use Medications Responsibly

The easy access and carefree use of over-the-counter and prescription drugs is a growing problem in our country—and I'm not referring to illegal drug use. Rather, I'm talking about the endless array of pain- and symptom-relieving medications that anyone can buy or have phoned in to the pharmacy with relative ease. The concept of taking a pill to relieve a physical or emotional symptom of discomfort is well entrenched in our culture. This is particularly alarming since many physical conditions could be easily addressed by making lifestyle changes.

Relying on a drug to fix what ails you—without addressing the underlying cause of those ailments—is very dangerous. It can lead to a complete abdication of responsibility for your health. Consider the message behind many of the drug commercials and advertisements today: "You don't have to give up the foods you love to avoid heartburn—just be sure to take 'X' acid controller when you eat your favorite foods." "Now you don't have to give in to your stress headaches, because prescription-strength 'X' pain relief is available over the counter." I've even seen a commercial for a digestive aid that said, "Why change your lifestyle when you can take a pill?"

Also disheartening are the countless brands of laxatives available—a sign that many people would rather pop a pill than eat the fruits, vegetables, and whole grains needed to stay healthy. The long row of symptom-suppressing cold medicines in our stores show Americans are willing to take anything for a cold, except perhaps a day off from work. You can know that the best care for a cold is drinking lots of fluids—fruit juices, chicken broth, and water—and getting plenty of rest. But it's just so appealing to think you can suppress the symptoms and keep up with your busy schedule.

Your body needs and deserves better treatment than squelching the symptom of an illness so you can frantically maintain a lifestyle—lack of rest, poor diet, and stress—that probably created an illness in the first place. When you constantly take the easy way out of discomfort, you forget that the best means of healing lies right inside of you, within your immune system. Your body's capacity to heal is miraculous. When you don't feel good, you need to listen to your body and address the root of what's making you sick. Many times this includes listening to your doctor and taking appropriate medications. But too often many people expect instant healing in the form of a pill. You must avoid this notion at all costs, especially if you want younger generations to get this. How can they when Mom's on Prozac, Dad's on Viagra, and they're on Ritalin?

Keep in mind that the way you address your simple digestive upsets, colds, and headaches can influence whether you get more serious illnesses in the future. For instance, indigestion is almost always a sign that you need to change your diet, eating environment, and the way you handle stress. Constipation is a dead giveaway that you aren't eating enough fruits, vegetables, and whole grains or drinking enough water. It also indicates a need for time and serenity around the all-important function of elimination. Frequent colds are a classic sign that your resistance is low and your immune system needs rebuilding. Round after round of antibiotics for a stubborn chest cold doesn't provide a long-term solution. Neither do symptom-stifling drugs. Headaches can be a sign of too much stress, too little sleep, a poor diet, or maybe too much caffeine. And all of these conditions are

161

things you can respond to proactively: You can increase your rest, intake of water and fresh fruits and vegetables, cut back on caffeine and junk food, and invest in and use a juicer.

These are just a few examples of the powerful choices you can make in response to the common aches and pains everyone experiences. The lure of drug advertisements and instant relief will always seem tempting. But you can maximize the curative effects of healthy lifestyle choices as a primary resource for healing and let medications be a secondary one.

Protect Yourself from the Sun

I'm the first to admit that soaking up the sun feels great and a *café au lait* tan can look very attractive. But sun worshipers—lying unprotected beneath the midday sun or frequenting the tanning booth—pay a high price with a substantially increased risk of skin cancer and the promise of prematurely aged skin. Yet many people continue to play Russian roulette with their health by pursuing the perfect tan.

Fortunately, deep, dark tans are less of a style, health, and beauty statement than they used to be, but even if they weren't, sometimes self-responsibility includes eschewing what's popular or fashionable. Also, you don't need to hide away from the great outdoors to avoid skin cancer these days. It's relatively easy to follow common sense guidelines regarding exposure to the sun.

First, don't frequent those ridiculous tanning booths. Invest in a serious sunscreen with sun protective factor, or SPF, of 30 or more—and apply it every day to exposed areas of the body. I find that keeping sunscreen next to my toothbrush on the bathroom counter helps me stay in the habit of using it daily. Also try to avoid all-out sun exposure between the peak hours of 10:00 A.M. to 3:00 P.M., especially during the summer months. Finally, it's a good idea to establish a relationship with a dermatologist for regular exams to check for changes in the size or shape of moles or any other irregularities of the skin.

162

Choose to Drive Safely

I'm passionate about the practice of safe, courteous driving, and in today's world it's basic to self-responsibility. In fact, depending, as most of us do, on a motor vehicle to get you where you need to go, it's a mistake not to consider your actions behind the driver's wheel as a measure of life expectancy and wellness.

When I started driving at age sixteen, my father gave me good advice: "Never forget a car can be a lethal weapon." Despite being a little overly dramatic, this remains a wise admonition. Cars do have the potential to maim and kill, and people die or are permanently disabled in car accidents every day.

One of the worst experiences in life is the feeling you get after suffering the results of your own bad judgment. It's a sense of being punished by your own hand or receiving a self-inflicted wound. Even more terrible is the price exacted of human life. There's no way to rewind the tape and play it back for different results; the consequences of a car accident will stay with you for a long time if you're fortunate enough to survive them.

There's no way to insure you'll never be in that situation, but the way you drive can definitely influence your odds. If you routinely screech into the gym parking lot after a hair-raising drive from the office through rush-hour traffic—while talking on a cell phone—you may as well skip the exercise in favor of prudent driving. The mistakes, misjudgments, and risks you indulge in going 60 miles an hour in a car have serious consequences. Anyone who's lost a loved one to a bad collision, or been in one themselves, knows the truth of this.

Self-responsible people wear seat belts and restrain their children in the backseat, leave ample time to get where they need to go without speeding, observe traffic laws, use turn indicators, don't tailgate, drive defensively, assume nothing so look both ways at every intersection, and respect the serious nature of driving and give it their full attention. They don't take chances with their own lives or the lives of others, either. They know they can choose a driving style that's life-threatening or life-enhancing—and they choose the latter.

The True Definition
of Healthcare

You've probably heard the terms "healthcare" and "health insurance" a lot these days because they're hot issues in both the political and media arenas. Healthcare and insurance are also things you don't want to be without but hope you never have to use.

However, the very word "healthcare" is somewhat of a misnomer— used to mean "sick care." By the time you enter the healthcare system, more often than not it's because you're . . . sick. And while "health insurance" implies the insurance of health, it means that if you're fortunate enough to get sick with a condition covered by your insurance policy, you'll get the benefit of medical treatment without losing your life savings in the process.

Imagine what those two terms could imply when taken with the most literal meanings. Healthcare would imply caring for and giving attention to health, and health insurance would imply actions and choices made in the interest of maintaining health and preventing disease. Who wouldn't benefit from changing the attitudes and perceptions about healthcare and health insurance? With soaring medical costs—and the increasing influence of insurance companies that dictate the parameters of medical treatment—no one can afford not to be proactive in this area of life.

Progress is being made in the healthcare industry toward education and preventive medicine. The concept of treating the whole person rather than a symptom of a disease is also beginning to take hold. However, as you consider the problems and limitations of the healthcare system, face your own part in it: Have you been a passive receiver of medical care rather than an active participant?

I have great hopes for the future of healthcare and modern medicine, and there are promising signs of change in the making. But the most important changes will be the ones you're willing to make as a healthcare consumer—the shift from a complacent, inactive patient to a self-empowered individual.

Self-responsibility is a great example of the power of choice you can make every day. In the same way that you choose to use your car carefully and keep it well-maintained, you can choose to treat your body with care. You can make the choice to drink lots of water, get the sleep you need, eat well, exercise regularly, and keep your emotional and spiritual house in order. Upon your yearly checkup, you can inform your doctor of the healthy choices you're making, ask for feedback on blood work or other routine tests ordered, and ask what additional lifestyle adjustments you should make to maintain optimal health. Make it clear that you consider your doctor to be one of many resources for continued good health, rather than an omniscient healer responsible for your well-being.

This scenario—which would be incredibly positive for patient and physician alike—is reasonable and well within the capabilities of any self-responsible adult. Imagine how the cost of healthcare would decrease if billions of dollars were not being spent on preventable, lifestyle-related diseases every year. You certainly would live in a different world with much higher expectations of good health if this example were reality. Even Laura Ingalls Wilder, who died in the year I was born, saw the truth of this: "There are those who persistently disobey the laws of health, which, being nature's laws, are also God's laws, and then when ill health comes, wonder why they should be compelled to suffer."

<hr />

However mean your life is, meet it and live it; do not shun it
and call it hard names. It is not so bad as you are.
The fault-finder will find fault even in paradise. Love your life.
HENRY DAVID THOREAU

Standing in line at the grocery store one Saturday, I overheard a woman complaining about the morning's rain even though the skies were starting to clear. "I just hate that the weather was bad today," this woman said. "Rain always ruins my weekend."

"Well," the clerk observed benignly, "we've had seven straight days of sunny weather. I guess one day of rain out of seven isn't too bad."

What a huge difference a positive mental outlook can make on something as innocuous as the weather! You really do have the choice to view the circumstances of life as "a glass half empty or a glass half full." Like the woman whose Saturday had been rained on, you can perceive events negatively. Or, like the grocery clerk, you can choose to look positively at the bright side of things. Ultimately, you're the only one who can control the direction of your thoughts.

Your ability to maintain a positive mental outlook depends a great deal on your maturity, state of emotional health, and sense of gratitude. Ten years ago my willingness to recognize and change my negative attitudes was much more limited than today; time and experience have since taught me that I can be the architect of my own happiness—if I'm willing to make the effort.

Another significant step toward having a positive mental outlook is abandoning the codependent mind-set that something outside of you or somebody besides you is responsible for your feelings. People who have made peace with their emotional issues tend to have a much more positive outlook on life; they don't perpetually choose the victim stance whenever life hits a rough patch.

Finally you can benefit from cultivating a sense of gratitude. In this age of discontent it's easy to lose perspective. But instead of continually adding up a list of grievances, you can focus on the abundance you have here and now.

Of course, there will be times when it's difficult to detect the silver lining in the dark clouds that come your way. I'm not suggesting that you put on a brave smile in response to real tragedy and misfortune, because there's definitely a time to grieve and feel despondent in this life. But how often do you give in to the fear-based attitudes that permeate our culture? How often do you dwell on the imagined shortcomings of your finances, career, or physical appearance? It's so easy to fall into negative thinking and then to let self-pity shade your perception of reality.

When I indulge in this behavior—and yes, sometimes I do—I turn to a trusted friend or one of my sisters as soon as I recognize what I'm doing, and I ask for help to regain a healthy perspective on things. Or I may simply remind myself that there are countless fellow human beings who would gladly exchange their problems for mine. The truth is when we're of sound body and mind, and our loved ones are safe, our troubles probably don't amount to much.

<hr />

If we had keen vision and feeling for all ordinary human life
it would be like hearing the grass grow and the squirrel's heart beat,
and we would die of the roar which lies on the other side of silence.
GEORGE ELIOT

I find it interesting that Mary Ann Evans, who wrote under the pen name of George Eliot, made this observation on human life during the 1800s, long before the advent of cellular phones, the nuclear age, and the Internal Revenue Service. One wonders what on earth could have been creating "the roar which lies on the other side of silence" in a time when people probably could listen to grass grow and hear a squirrel's heart beat.

When a pattern of chaos and stress takes its toll on your quality of life, it usually means a measure of self and time management have fallen by the wayside. In a world that thrives on chaos and considers stress to be normal, you can't expect to be rescued from the disarray of your own making. You have to identify your tendency to overwork and overschedule, and make changes. Unfortunately it can take a nervous breakdown before some people decide to get out of life's fast lane.

Being self-responsible in the face of the stress and strain of modern life doesn't mean living in perfect balance. I don't know anyone who can do this, myself included. However, each of us has our own warning light that comes on when the symptoms of stress build up. Sometimes it comes in the form of a physical symptom like sleeplessness or a big red pimple that pops up out of nowhere. The warning can also be a familiar issue in life that keeps coming back to haunt

167

you, like a relationship, or money problem. Self-responsibility means choosing to address these warnings rather than ignore them. And it means taking the initiative to smooth out the rough edges of our lifestyles, whether it's the fashionable thing to do or not.

To embrace the virtue of self-responsibility is as much a lifelong endeavor as any other component of a healthy lifestyle. The basics you've been reading about are simple and practical but not necessarily easy.

In fact today's world frequently makes a virtue out of victimhood. This is painfully obvious in the prevalence of lawsuits, the reluctance of people to assume responsibility for reasonable healthcare; and the refusal to confront the consequences of lifestyle choices like smoking, drug use, and sexual promiscuity. You'll be tempted to play the victim in our culture—and for anyone who values the gift of life, this is a trap to be on guard against and to avoid. As Kathleen Tierney Andrus says: "To wait for someone else, or to expect someone else to make my life richer, or fuller, or more satisfying, puts me in a constant state of suspension."

Self-responsibility as a way of life is encouraging, empowering, ultimately satisfying, and will enhance your life immeasurably.

The Power of Choice

Things you can do every day to impact your well-being

- **Think about the choices you can make to change things you control.** What actions could you take to make your life a better one? Write down in separate categories what's right and what's wrong with your life. Give yourself a pat on the back for the good things. Now look at the WRONG column. Divide those issues into "Things I Have No Control Over" and "Things I Can Change." What's in the WRONG column that you may be bringing on yourself? What could you do daily to live a healthier and more fulfilling life? Remember, the intent to be self-responsible is the first step toward achieving it.

- **Stock up on fruits and vegetables twice a week so you can make the good choices essential to a healthy lifestyle.** To start, open your refrigerator and take an unflinching look at what's there now. Do you have an abundant supply of fresh foods to choose from, or are you staring at a lot of processed convenience foods?

- **Resolve to treat your body's symptoms with respect and tender care rather than a quick fix.** Abusing medications may be commonplace in our culture, but it doesn't have to be in your home. Take a good hard look at your medicine cabinet. Are you unconsciously abusing over-the-counter remedies in lieu of taking care of yourself? Remember: Pain is only a symptom, and sometimes a headache or stomachache are the only way your body can get your attention.

169

- **Evaluate your relationship with your doctor(s).** Are you working with him or her to care for your health, or are you dependent and needy? Remember that doctors are human beings with the same hopes, fears, and mortality as the rest of us. They can get just as sick as we can, and they too are vulnerable. Consider your doctor part of your team for good health, just as you would consider an accountant part of your financial team. Show yourself and your doctor some respect by listening to his or her advice, and doing what you can on your own.

- **Be willing to stretch the concept of health insurance and healthcare.** When I buy nutritional supplements or go to the massage therapist or chiropractor and pay those fees myself, I consider it a form of real health insurance. What investments could you be making in your healthcare right now that aren't covered by insurance? Preventive maintenance is the key to good health and isn't a luxury. Sometimes it just boils down to your priorities in life. How good do you want to feel today, a year from now, or ten years from now?

- **Remember that self-responsibility does not mean self-blame.** Sometimes things will go wrong with your body—or your life, and doing the best you can while working with what you've been given is a great achievement in its own right. Self-responsibility is not an insurance policy that guarantees good health, but it's the best investment you can make.

Eight

Your Relationship
to Others

We cannot live only for ourselves.
A thousand fibers connect us
with our fellow men; and among
those fibers as sympathetic threads,
our actions run as causes, and
they come back to us as effects.

HERMAN MELVILLE

The year I started this book began with two sudden trips to Montana in the bitter cold of winter. My Uncle Huby had been in declining health, and a series of strokes finally landed him in a nursing home near the house where he and Aunt Lois had lived since retirement. Something inside told me I'd better visit this dear uncle, whom I'd not seen in several years.

When I called Aunt Lois about coming up, I asked her if I should bring my fiddle.

"Oh, Ruth," she said, "please do that. Huby would love it."

So I packed some pictures, warm clothes, and my fiddle, and off I went for a long weekend in Hamilton, Montana.

On a cold but sunny January day, I stood before dear Uncle Huby and Aunt Lois in the dining hall of a nursing home and played for them—classical melodies, bluegrass tunes, old church hymns. As I played I remembered how I hadn't really known Uncle Huby or Aunt Lois well until I was twelve and our family moved from Illinois to California.

Huby, who was the firstborn child of my Grandpa and Grandma Huber, and my mother's older brother by eighteen years, had seemed far away to us when we were in the Midwest. Then, at our new home near Los Angeles, Uncle Huby and Aunt Lois lived just an hour away. Spending time with them was one of the best things about that move.

I'll never forget the fabulous day, shortly after our arrival in California, when they treated our family to Disneyland. They wanted to make up for all the birthdays and holidays missed when we lived in the Midwest; this would be just the beginning of their doing so in a hundred different ways.

The Uncle Huby I'd known then was a tall man with a unique amble to his walk. He'd inherited Grandpa Huber's chiseled good looks and Grandma Huber's stern sense of propriety. He'd learned to play the violin when he was a boy and taught lessons during his college years. With that connection, he was always intrigued with the music my sisters and I played. In fact, he and Aunt Lois never missed a recital or school concert; when it came time for me to get a truly fine instrument, they loaned my parents some of the money with a low rate of interest and flexible payment schedule. They were thrilled to be able to help my other sisters in a similar fashion.

Now, decades later in Montana, I was playing for them once again. My music and this trip were an expression to my uncle at the end of his life, certainly a testament of my love for him, but more than that, too—a reflection of the investment Uncle Huby made in me from my awkward age of 12, through the school years, and into adulthood. How I'd always felt Huby's and Lois's interest and enjoyment. Now I felt the weight of their 58-year marriage. They sat together: Huby in his wheelchair, Lois beside him, holding his hand, tears streaming down each of their faces. I knew Uncle Huby was near the end of his life, and he knew I was there to say goodbye.

Two weeks later he was gone. And two weeks later I would be in Montana again with my fiddle, this time to play "Amazing Grace" for his memorial service.

Though I'd just returned home from Montana and was profoundly grateful I'd been able to honor Uncle Huby while he was living, I'd felt strongly about honoring my uncle upon death with the music he loved so much, too. I realized what a grandfather-like figure he'd been for me and my sisters. I barely remember Grandpa Huber, because he died when I was quite young, but Uncle Huby filled that gap. He took me fishing and told me stories. He was interested in my musical dreams and supported them. He was so kind, very wise, and made a huge difference in my life.

What if I hadn't listened to that feeling about visiting sooner rather than later?

When we get to heaven I doubt that the cars, the clothes, and the bank account balances of this life will be very important. I think we'll know the worst and best of what we've done with our lives. We'll understand that in the final analysis our human capacity to love will be what's mattered most; ultimately our contribution will be judged by our connections to each other, not the material things left behind.

All of us yearn to have meaning, and I believe we find that meaning by connecting with God and our fellow human beings. Nothing substitutes for this need or replaces it—not a quest for the perfect body, ageless face, work we've done, or achievements made. We can only find meaning in our experiences with each other and the knowledge that whatever differences we may have, we share the same destiny. We'll all experience joy and sorrow, communion and loneliness, birth and death. These are essential threads that tie us together.

The world is so empty if one thinks only of mountains, rivers and cities;
but to know someone here and there who thinks and feels with us,
and who, though distant, is close to us in spirit,
this makes the earth for us an inhabited garden.

JOHANN WOLFGANG GOETHE

When I was just eight years old, a family moved across the street and up two houses from us in Decatur, Illinois, and I found my first best friend. Her name was Virginia, and she was four years older than I, which made the friendship seem all the more special. We became inseparable playmates and shared many adventures.

Five years later, when my family packed up and moved to California, I cried all the way across Kansas. I was sure my life would never be the same.

I was right. I never had another playmate like Virginia. But I had begun the lifelong continuum of making new friends.

In California, developing friendships was difficult for me until I met a girl named Jackie in my junior high school. Jackie was Jewish and different from anyone I'd ever known, and we developed a very special friendship. She invited me to her home on many occasions, once to share the Passover Seder with her family, and it was this wonderful occasion that introduced me to the beauty of the Jewish faith, the unique qualities of the chosen people, to folk dancing and spicy Yiddish expressions. My life is the richer for it.

When I started college, I met a fellow violinist named Nancy who proved pivotal in my life. Three years into my major of music at California State University, Nancy swept me up in her enthusiasm to go across country and audition for the Juilliard School of Music. If not for her, I don't think I'd have gathered the courage or taken that plunge on my own.

I'll never forget the day we arrived in New York City either. Bleary-eyed from taking the red-eye flight but exhilarated beyond measure, I simply couldn't get over the sight of the Manhattan skyline at daybreak. By evening, Nancy and I and the two other friends who also came to audition sat on the floor of a tiny studio apartment and ate the best pizza I'd ever tasted, exclaiming over the experience we were just beginning. There's nothing like the sound and feel of a late summer evening in New York City from the seventh floor of an old apartment building with the windows wide open—and once again I knew my life would never be the same.

I was right. Nancy and I were both accepted by Juilliard, and we shared an apartment in New York for three years.

During that time I developed a close friendship with another violinist named Wendy, who joined Nancy and me when we moved uptown to a larger apartment. Wendy and I had a great deal in common and during the Juilliard years and the time shortly after, we shared the joys and miseries of being twenty-something. We fell in love, out of love, moved, started jobs, changed jobs—and through it all we knew each other's greatest hopes and fears. I can't imagine how I would have negotiated my New York years without her.

Wendy eventually moved to Austria to pursue her lifelong dream of living and playing in an orchestra in Europe. But we've kept in touch with an occasional visit and volumes of letters, cards, and notes; I always feel a special surge of happiness when I open my mailbox to find an airmail letter from Austria.

I can't imagine life without Wendy (who remains one of the few close friends with whom I can share anything). I'm glad I don't have to, either, because whatever deficits have been in my life I count my friendships as one of my greatest successes. From my childhood in Decatur, Illinois, to today in Nashville, Tennessee, the friends who have resonated with me as kindred spirits, have helped me embrace life with a fearless curiosity. They've also made an indelible mark on me as a woman, an artist, and a human being.

No doubt by now you're thinking of your own friends: the people you love and who love you in return, the people who dot the landscape of your years and mark like milestones where you've been and how far you've come. They remind you of the things you never would have done or never could have lived through without them.

Scan through all of them in your mind. Scanning your memories for shared moments with friends is never a wasted effort, because what a privilege it is to have a friend, what a great investment with a priceless return. Think of how your friends have sustained you, molded you, and influenced your path in life—probably as much as your blood relatives, if not more so.

While there are many different levels of friendships, all of them have value. The friends who give your life the most meaning are usually the ones you can count on one hand. These are the friends who know you intimately, understand how you operate, accept the good and bad in you, and love you unconditionally.

My closest friends share little in common, except that each one would drop everything to be there for me in a crisis, and I would do the same for them. These are friendships that developed out of shared interests and grew naturally to include mutual respect and shared experiences.

They're friends like Sherry, whom I met a couple of years before moving to Nashville. Sherry was looking for a fiddler to open a show for Tanya Tucker. I accepted the job with trepidation because I was still a novice fiddler, just making the transition from classical music to country and bluegrass. But I played the show with Sherry and was almost immediately taken in as a full-time band member. The exploits and escapades of my years with Sherry and the Stonewall Junction Band are enough to fill the pages of another book. What fun we had and what great music we played! What an influence this was on my life too, leading directly to my decision to move to Nashville, where country music was really happening.

In the years since that move, I've never lost touch with Sherry, and when we visit each other it's as if we've never been apart. We are friends for life, and we both know it.

Friendships at this level carry a unique momentum. They require an investment of time but need not be forced in order to grow. Yet because time has become such a strained commodity in today's world, friendships frequently suffer. Long-distance friendships, especially, can fall through the cracks without regular care and feeding. But even friends who live in the same time zone and area code can fall by the wayside if you let them. The result can impact the quality and meaning of day-to-day life.

I've fallen into this trap more than once but am grateful for friendships resilient enough to bounce back. This didn't happen on its own however. Relationships need to be nurtured as intently as you would nurture your body with food and rest. A well-timed phone call or spur-of-the-moment get-together can pump new life into a neglected friendship with amazing results.

One of my dear friends, Lee, used to meet me for sushi once a week before she had children. For a few memorable years we enjoyed frequent phone calls and weekly engagements of one sort or another. Then our respective lives and lifestyles changed. Today we have to be more deliberate about staying in touch and getting together, so we take turns being the one who makes the effort to connect. But connect we do, and it's always wonderfully rewarding. We fall back into our easy way of relating and confiding without any hesitation.

Lee can look me straight in the eye, say, "You have a problem here," and I'll know she is right. The fact that we don't see each other as often as we used to doesn't make me trust her any less. Our

177

mutual regard is based on the safety and ease that comes with a solid friendship.

Another good friend, Kathy, has been a fixture in my life ever since I moved to Nashville. As a fellow musician and gifted singer, Kathy has shared some unique experiences with me, both onstage and off. She's seen me through a difficult romantic breakup, and I've walked with her through the dregs of a doomed marriage. She's the only person (other than my Aunt Cathy), whom I've ever known to feel the same passion for dogs that I do.

When I was still a night owl playing club dates as a fiddler, Kathy and I used to go for walks. On balmy Nashville summer nights we'd discuss the ins and outs of the music business. Then I started to teach and train in the early morning hours, and our midnight walks came to an end.

Despite conflicting schedules, we maintain our friendship by meeting over a cup of coffee. If we can't do so in person, we talk on the phone—and those phone calls have sustained me through many challenging times.

Do you see or talk to the friends you can count on one hand often enough? It's easy to lose the constancy of a great friendship as you get busier and older, but it doesn't have to be an inevitable loss. When you purposefully invest time and effort in your dearest friendships, the payback is unbelievable. As Anne Wilson Schaef, the author of *Escape from Intimacy*, says, "It is not possible to live a rich, full life without friends. I have to be one to have one."

<hr />

*Fatherly and motherly hearts often beat warm and wise in the breasts
of bachelor uncles and maiden aunts; and it is my private opinion
that these worthy creatures are a beautiful provision of nature
for the cherishing of other people's children.*

LOUISA MAY ALCOTT

I'll never forget the day I first laid eyes on my dad's youngest sister, my wonderful Aunt Cathy. I was eight years old, living in Decatur, Illinois, and waiting impatiently for this aunt to arrive for a long visit.

She was driving out to see us from Albuquerque, New Mexico, where she lived and worked as a nurse. My father had a picture of her in her nurse's uniform, and I already felt I knew this pretty woman.

After an interminable wait, she pulled up alongside the curb in front of our house and stepped out of a big, green bomb of a station wagon. She came to the front door, all tall and slender and beautiful, with the sleekest ponytail and brightest red lipstick I'd ever seen. On one arm she held three stuffed animals—dogs!—one for each of us girls. I fell head over heels in love with Aunt Cathy that day and instantly connected with her in a way that never faltered or changed for the rest of her life.

My aunt moved to Decatur shortly thereafter, to work as a nurse and continue her training as a nurse-anesthesiologist. This gave me many opportunities to get to know and love her. Our lives became intwined in a special way. There was nothing better than going over to visit Aunt Cathy at her apartment. We made Toll House cookies together and invariably ate too many. She took me to wonderful movies like *My Fair Lady* and *Mary Poppins*. And going to the movies with Aunt Cathy always included a stop at the candy store, so I'd come home from our special dates with stars in my eyes and chocolate on my fingers. When my aunt dated the handsome bachelor farmer who lived next door to us, she became even more intriguing to me.

When my family made the move to California, it was particularly wrenching to be separated from this special aunt. But the investment she had made in my life carried a substantial weight. A lifeline resonated between us even as our lives changed. She married the bachelor next door and had a child. I went away to school and started a career. We kept in touch with phone calls, letters, and an occasional visit—and when I moved to Nashville the visits became more frequent.

Over the years I watched my aunt lose her youthful vitality and relinquish some of her dreams. I watched her shift her focus to her daughter's needs and indulge her passion for animals. Her weight fluctuated, and she had bouts with depression. As an adult I came to understand that life had been hard on Aunt Cathy. But through it all, the beautiful person she was never changed. Her nonjudgmental acceptance of

179

others made her safe to confide in. She had a sense of humor that never disappointed. Her steady Christian faith was like a welcoming beacon through good times and bad, and her compassion for people and animals was inspiring.

During the last year of her life, I visited Aunt Cathy every chance I could. The seriousness of her diagnosis made each moment we shared more significant. She recalled old family stories that helped me understand the legacy of my father's parents. I promised to renew my relationship with her daughter, my cousin, Andrea. Our conversations about the passions we shared for everything from Jane Austen movies to animal welfare accelerated like a tape pushed to fast forward. How grateful I am today that I could be with her so much in her final year.

A few times during that year, as I psyched myself up for another drive to Illinois, people asked me, "How can you make these trips out of town with so much going on in your life?" This was a reasonable question, considering the extra projects I'd taken on, not the least of which was my wedding. But I was crystal clear about my devotion to my aunt. It was born the day I first met her, as she handed me a cute, stuffed dog, rooted in thirty years of knowing that she loved me no matter what I was up to, or how badly I was running my life. My devotion, in turn, was a tribute to the investment she'd made in me every year of my life.

Despite all the pain that can be passed down through the generations, there's nothing like the ties that bind family together. Whatever you receive, both the good and the bad becomes a blueprint for your own life, and you need to celebrate the relationships that are most dear.

Even the relationships that don't come easily can provide a unique legacy. You truly learn about yourself through the connections you have with others. You can glean so much from the ones who have lived before you, and you can learn from their mistakes and gain from their wisdom.

Anne Fremantle, the author of *A Treasury of Early Christianity*, reminds, "We cannot fail to meet the same problems as did our forefathers, and learning their answers may help us to act upon them as intelligently as they did, and may even, perhaps, teach us to avoid making the same mistakes."

Do you see how you can sense the impact and the sanctity of your own life when it's set against the backdrop of your family's? When I look through photos of Aunt Cathy as a young woman, I see myself in the tilt of her head and the way she crossed her long legs. When I look at my youngest sister, Erin, I see the purity of the Huber line in the structure of her body and bones in her face. When I look at the picture on my bedroom wall of my father's mother, who died before I was born, I see a young girl dressed a little like a gypsy, playing the violin. I've often felt a part of her—an obvious kindred spirit—lives on in me.

The feeling of being part of something bigger and deeper than you are alone can give you a sense of the eternal picture. Ultimately, that's a picture only God can see and control. But if you know in your heart, through your ties to family and other human beings, that your journey is part of that picture and that it matters, you have a different way of approaching life.

My Aunt Cathy had her problems and shortcomings, but her legacy transcends whatever struggles she had in this life. During her final months, she reminded me in a hundred different ways to carefully consider my own legacy. That was her last and greatest gift to me and one I hold close each day.

Do you have an aunt, uncle, or other relative who has made a difference in your life? Do you stay in touch with them? In this time when so many families are fragmented, you need more than ever to reach out to something solid and real. A letter or phone call can open the path of communication in a heartbeat. Snapshots of day-to-day life can update a relative with very few words and are easy to pop in the mail with a short note.

Here's another idea—what are you doing over your next vacation? Could you include a visit to someone in the family whom you love but haven't seen in a while? The wealth in these gestures goes both ways. I had a rich and satisfying visit with my Aunt Lois when I traveled to Montana twice the year Uncle Huby died. Then she gifted me with her presence at my wedding nine months later, which thrilled me to no end. For the rest of my life I'll be able to leaf through my wedding pictures and see Aunt Lois enjoying that celebration with me.

If you're unable to see your loved ones, do you ever think about the remarkable character traits that run through your extended family? The way an uncle spoke a certain phrase, or the way an aunt set her lips together to express an emotion? Do you know what quirks of nature you came by honestly because they run in the family? My great-grandmother on my father's side made and drank coffee that would hold a fork upright. While I don't make my coffee that strong, I do love it robust. It makes me smile to think of this simple pleasure that I share with my great-grandmother who lived well into her nineties.

What favorite foods and recipes have you inherited from your ancestors? Can you duplicate those today for your own family? It's fun to carry on old traditions—and many of them center around the foods we enjoy on holidays or during certain seasons of the year. Aunt Cathy always had a stash of *Pepparkakar* cookies in her house around Christmas time. I'll always remember how great these cookies tasted dunked in coffee, and I can know the recipe for this hard, sweet treat came from a long line of cookie bakers in her mother's Swedish family.

These nuances of personality and tradition are as important now as ever to remember and pass along to future generations. Up until fifty years ago multigenerational living was commonplace—three generations would sit down to a Sunday dinner together every week. Today, as families split up and move around more often, the sense of connectedness from one generation to the next has become more difficult to feel. The rich heritage of a family line is a sad thing to lose, and that loss fragments our society.

That special sense of family connection is what I felt the night before my September 1996 wedding at age 39. The rehearsal dinner over and house empty, I pulled out my wedding dress to move over some fastening hooks. For some reason I'd waited until the last minute to do this. Suddenly, as I stood before that beautiful, freshly steamed and pressed handmade dress—the one my Grandma Huber designed and sewed to wear at her own wedding 83 years earlier—I knew I wasn't alone. I felt the spirit of my grandma in the room.

Eighty-three years and a few months earlier, my grandma Lulu Jabusch (soon to be Huber) probably fussed with the last-minute details of that very same dress. She was a much younger bride in a much simpler time, yet no doubt as tired and excited as I was—as most brides are. She knew she was on the brink of a different kind of life. My eyes filled with tears as I thought of this and worked with her dress, amazed at how tightly she'd sewn the hooks to the fabric. *Did she have any idea that a grandchild might wear her wedding gown long after she was gone? Could she have known the intimate gift of her legacy?* I felt the lightning speed with which generation follows generation swirl around me and experienced a pang of regret for all the things I never knew about my grandma. Then I had a rush of gratitude for feeling as close to her as I did in that moment.

Every person has a special place in this world and a story to tell. What dear relatives in your life right now can help you explore this kind of buried treasure? What you learn from the lives of those who came before you will add to the meaning of your own.

<hr>

(To) take something from yourself, to give to another, that is humane and gentle and never takes away as much comfort as it brings again.

THOMAS MOORE

When you pick up a newspaper or watch the evening news, it can sometimes be hard to feel connected to your neighbors and community. It's easy to develop a hard shell around the heart and turn your eyes away from human suffering that seems to have no purpose and no end. But if you retreat more and more into a high-security home or sterile world of computers and television, you only become increasingly removed from human need.

This is a challenge of our time and new chapter in human development that you're among one of the first generations to see daily and in living color. You know this challenge: One person's inhumanity to another—incomprehensible acts of violence and hate that maim and kill for no reason. You see children lose their innocence earlier and

183

become part of the problem sooner. Something clicks off between the brain and the soul when you witness the aftermath of a plane crash, a senseless murder, or some other terrible disaster on a daily basis. You become numb and desensitized to bad things, and you forget that the human spirit has the potential to transcend the tragedies of life.

It's easy to feel overwhelmed when considering the plight of the human condition. A natural response is to want to crawl back into your shell like a turtle. But the burning desire to get up, brush yourself off, and try again is also part of being human. Every person is born with the ability to make a contribution. The Holy Spirit works inside you to help you be better than yourself. No matter how hopeless things look, you always have the ability to affect another life in a positive way. The random kindness you give and receive could be your truest purpose in this life, one of the best reasons for getting out of bed in the morning.

You won't find the inspiration for acts of kindness, patience, and compassion on the six o'clock news—at least not very often. So where can you look and where do you start? How about by practicing kindness as a way of life with everyone you encounter?

I was standing in line at the bank one day and witnessed such kindness in action. A fragile, silver-haired woman was at a teller window trying to take care of a money problem. Just that morning she had withdrawn five hundred dollars in cash—probably her spending money for the month—and somehow mislaid her wallet a few hours later. She was alone and upset, frail, and a bit hard of hearing. I felt the frustration and unhappiness of her situation with real regret. The bank teller, a young man, patiently listened and helped this lady above and beyond the call of duty. He asked if she needed help canceling her credit cards. He offered to get her a chair so she could sit down. Another woman who had just finished her transactions stopped to commiserate. Unfolding was human compassion and kindness at work, and it made me feel better about the world for the rest of the day.

Instances of kindness that stretch the capacity of the human heart come in all shapes and sizes. Sometimes they save lives and other times they just save a day. Think about ones you've seen recently. For instance, have you ever left the house in a snit some morning—really on the wrong foot—only to have your day completely turned around because someone treated you kindly? A man in a truck smiled and waved you into the traffic lane in front of him, helping you get to work on time. A child flung his arms around your neck and planted a sloppy kiss on your cheek to transform your attitude. The lady at the bank window greeted you with genuine respect and made you feel a little better about yourself. Like manna from heaven, these small gestures of kindness, given without an agenda or expectation, are valuable to both the giver and the receiver.

During the rollercoaster ride of the year I married, I had the good fortune to receive gestures of kindness on a regular basis. In July, after a particularly grueling trip to Illinois to see Aunt Cathy in the hospital, I came home to find my Akita, JoJo, in a mysterious decline. He'd lost weight while I was gone, refused to eat, and moped around, listless and unhappy. After a week of tempting him with countless treats and hovering over him to no avail, John and I drove him to the Veterinary Hospital at the University of Tennessee in Knoxville. A woman named Dr. Anderson looked at him and shook her head, fearing JoJo had a terminal illness. As we made arrangements to check him into intensive care, I was overwhelmed with tears. I buried my head in JoJo's furry neck and just broke down. Dr. Anderson reached for some tissues and sent the assisting student out of the examination room. With an unusual degree of empathy she allowed me to hold JoJo and compose myself.

In that wretched moment she exercised kindness and on some level invested herself in helping JoJo. The week that followed was very hard. I had to return to Nashville to resume work and wedding preparations. But the kindness and compassion Dr. Anderson exhibited went a long way toward giving me some peace of mind. I was confident that JoJo was in loving hands and knew this doctor would exhaust all possibilities for a cure. She had reinforced my hope that good things could come out of even the darkest hour.

In the end, they did. JoJo amazed everyone and made a remarkable recovery. Dr. Anderson had traced his problem to a chemical imbalance in the adrenal system, stabilized by a tiny dose of daily medicine. JoJo was put on the road to recovery, and I'm convinced that happy ending was largely influenced by our doctor's ability to care deeply.

Little miracles like these spring directly from God's love working through people. When you understand and receive the love of God, you in turn can love generously. In a world that so often appears, as the cliché says, to be going to hell in a handbasket, it's imperative to exercise your ability to love one another at every opportunity.

When was the last time someone did something nice for you out of the blue? When was the last time you witnessed a kind gesture from a distance? How did these moments make you feel about yourself and about life? Chances are, you misted over for a minute. Perhaps you felt like reaching out yourself. There's no way to judge the potential of one kind gesture. The loving energy involved in it ripples out in countless invisible waves, and once initiated, it takes on a beautiful life of its own.

The small things you do for fellow human beings might be the greatest things you do in life. Letting someone who's harried and rushed get in front of you in the checkout line of the grocery store. Helping an elderly person negotiate a flight of stairs or accompanying him or her across a busy street. Handing a homeless person the grilled chicken sandwich you just picked up at the drive-through restaurant.

There's a beautiful tradition in the Jewish faith of bestowing an act of kindness, called a *mitzvah*. The rule of the *mitzvah* is that it must remain anonymous. The person who receives it never knows who it came from. The person who gives it never tells a soul. It's an exercise in generosity that circumvents the ego. Imagine what the world would be like if everyone learned to bestow kindness in this selfless manner on a daily basis.

To laugh often and love much, to win the respect of intelligent persons and the affection of children;. . . to appreciate beauty; to find the best in others; to give one's self; . . . to know even one life breathed easier because you have lived, this is to have succeeded.

RALPH WALDO EMERSON

When you make yourself vulnerable and reach out—whether to a relative, friend, or complete stranger—you make a connection with the human adventure that began in the Garden of Eden. There, the agony and the ecstasy of humanity was born. Today, you experience that same agony and ecstasy. So much in life is out of your control and beyond your power to influence. But your life has meaning, purpose, and worth as you connect with another. This is one of the great gifts of life.

When my Aunt Cathy passed away in the fall of 1996, the small farming community where she lived (a place just outside of the Illinois town where I grew up), reached out with support and kindness. I'd spent a busy week helping plan the funeral with family members arriving and the general busyness that surrounds a death. The generosity and thoughtfulness of the people who knew and loved my aunt touched me deeply. They brought comfort and food, provided lodging and airport runs, and gave flowers as a testament to the memory of my aunt and a reflection of those who loved her.

In all the acts of kindness, one stands out in my mind. One of my aunt's best friends searched me out after the memorial service and acknowledged my pain and loss in a subtle but beautiful way. During the reception back at the house, with people milling about, talking, eating, and drinking, I was experiencing a common feeling after a death—the surreal expectation that my aunt could just walk in the front door at any moment. Sitting in the gentle roar of people visiting, I looked up to see my aunt's friend. She fixed her eyes on mine and held me for a moment with a glance of knowing and compassion. My eyes filled with tears and my heart felt huge and tight. I could barely swallow the bite of food I'd just taken.

Without saying a word, this dear friend had expressed to me, "I know what you've lost. I know how much you meant to her. I know this loss cannot be eased. I grieve with you."

In a way I can't explain, with nothing more than a tender glance, she comforted me and eased my broken heart. More than any other person I connected with in the aftermath of that dreadful week, this woman touched me at the center of my being. She showed me that while there's

187

no way to relieve the grief of bereavement, the efforts of one human being to comfort another can help salve the raw edge of loss.

There's no way to measure your investment in others or the return on that investment. There's no RDA for kindness and connecting either. But your life yearns for meaning as much as your body craves food and water. To feel the eternal pulse of the human spirit is to be in touch with yourself and with God. Your ability to warm another's heart and experience this essence of humanity might just be the fullest measure of your life.

The Power of Choice

Things you can do every day to impact your well-being

- **Write an informal account of your life to pass on to those who love you.** In her final year my Aunt Cathy compiled a list of family memories for her daughter, Andrea—stories about her mother and father, the unique characteristics of her grandmother and aunts, and other odds and ends like songs, poetry, and prayers she'd grown up with. I was grateful that all those special memories hadn't been lost or wasted. Our personal histories can provide a wealth of insight and wisdom to those we leave behind. Consider recording the outstanding memories in your life as a gift for those you love.

- **Create or help preserve the rich story of your life and your ancestors's.** If you're like me, you probably have wonderful photographs buried in shoe boxes in the corner of a closet somewhere. Take the time to unearth them, then make some beautiful photo albums by spending a rainy afternoon poring over and organizing the best pictures you have. Keep these photo albums on your coffee table or some other accessible place in your home to enjoy the pictures and share them with friends.

- **Create a gallery of family pictures on a wall in your house.** See how far back in your family tree you can go with photographs that bring your ancestors to life. Do you have some great old photos large enough to frame and hang on a wall? Photo reproduction and restoration is inexpensive and easy to do with today's technology. Make copies to send to siblings or other relatives who

189

would also cherish them. Then get them professionally mounted and framed.

• **Rediscover how good it feels and what little time and effort it really takes to brighten the life of a dear friend or relative with a letter.** Although letter writing has become a lost art in our culture, even the most jaded among us is thrilled at the arrival of a personal note in the mail. Once you start, you'll find how fulfilling and fun it is to write—and receive—a letter. It's also contagious. But the best way to receive a letter is to send one. Make a cup of tea, sit down with some pretty stationery and a really great pen, and write a dear friend or relative.

• **Drive with courtesy and make it a goal to positively affect someone else's life each time you get behind the steering wheel.** It's one of the easiest ways in this increasingly uncivil world to practice simple kindness toward people you don't know and may never see again. It also takes so little time to let someone pull into the lane in front of you, or smile and acknowledge a driver who has gifted you with such courtesy.

Nine

Honoring the Spirit

And I have felt a presence that disturbs me
with the joy
Of elevated thoughts; a sense sublime
Of something far more deeply interfused,
Whose dwelling is the light of setting suns,
And the round ocean and the living air,
And the blue sky, and in the mind of man:
A motion and a spirit, that impels
All thinking things, all objects of all thoughts,
And rolls through all things.

WILLIAM WORDSWORTH,
"LINES COMPOSED . . . ABOVE TINTERN ABBEY"

There's a place in Nashville called Radnor Lake with a loveliness that's perpetually changing. This state-protected wildlife area encompasses more than one thousand acres of hills, woods, and trails surrounding a tranquil eighty-acre lake.

During the hot, muggy days of summer, you can disappear into the woods to enjoy cooler temperatures, provided by the shade of the forest and breeze coming off the water.

Autumn brings an artist's palette of color, as the leaves turn gold, red, and orange—all reflected against the lake. Later in the fall, those leaves cover the paths, and new vistas appear behind bare tree branches.

Winter has its own breathtaking beauty. In January, the trails are covered with freshly chipped, recycled Christmas trees, blanketing the hard ground with a springy, fragrant greenery that adds pleasure to bleak winter walks.

Then, just as the gray, cold days feel like they'll never end, hints of spring break through. The air gradually warms up, the days lengthen, and finally tiny green leaves begin to appear as the redbud and dogwood trees spread out their blossoms. Mother Nature's beautiful cycle continues, month after month, season after season, and year after year.

I've walked the trails and hiked the hills of Radnor Lake for fifteen years and never grown tired of it. I go there with friends, family, and clients every chance I get, but what I love most is going there alone. When I walk into those woods by myself I'm immediately aware of God's presence.

I can remember as a young girl wandering off to a quiet place in the woods during my family's frequent camping trips and feeling that I wasn't alone. Now, as then, it's partly eerie, partly comforting. My brain stops its analyzing, my ego retreats, and I find myself more willing to listen.

Spiritual contemplation is easy to forego in the face of the more pressing matters of modern life. I know, because I did this for years. But today I understand that there isn't a concern that cannot be at least partially addressed by retreating from the distractions of the world to a place of silence. Like most of the answers I have found in my life, this understanding came to me the hard way.

My road to faith and embracing God has been a rocky one. For many years I didn't pray or go to church. Today, as much as I love certain passages of Scripture, especially the Psalms, I'm not a great scholar of the Bible. I get caught up in my daily routine and neglect my spirit more often than I care to admit. But time and time again, as life's circumstances alternately bring me to my knees or to my feet with arms raised to heaven, I'm grateful to feel certain of God's love. It's, frankly, a relief to feel a part of something greater than myself.

—∞—

> *Make your ego porous. Will is of little importance,*
> *complaining is nothing, fame is nothing. Openness,*
> *patience, receptivity, solitude is everything.*
> RAINER MARIA RILKE

One of my earliest recollections of childhood is going to church on Sundays. I can close my eyes and visualize the Presbyterian church in Decatur and the Sunday school classrooms where I learned about Jesus and his disciples. My mother, a church organist and choir director for as long as I can remember, often had a job in a different church than the one our family attended, so we were always involved in two churches.

As I grew up I understood that going to church was something we did on Sunday. When we sat down to dinner as a family, one of us girls would say grace before the meal. As soon as my skills on the violin allowed, Mother had me accompany her choir. I performed often in the churches we attended over the years—sometimes the opportunities were rewarding, but mostly nerve-racking. As I think back

193

on all of that, I'm grateful I was raised in a family that went to church on Sunday and gave thanks before the evening meal.

Now I realize much of what I experienced as a child was simply going through motions. I embraced the basic tenets of Christianity but had no concept of the true meaning of grace, redemption, and faith.

When I was 14 years old, on the verge of being confirmed in our church, I had my first experience with death. One of my best junior high school friends, a bright and lovely girl named Theresa Molitor, was killed while riding her bike after school. She'd unwittingly set out to cross a busy street, right in front of an oncoming car. I'll never forget the scene around the lockers where we all met before class or the grim expressions on the teachers' faces as we tried to digest the fact that Theresa was dead.

Whatever faith I had in God was shattered that day. I simply couldn't reconcile the God I understood to be great and good with this tragic turn of events. Through the days and weeks following that terrible accident, I retreated into my own numb world. I was the only member of my confirmation class to choose not to be confirmed. Although I continued to have a church life, I became emotionally and spiritually unavailable. There's no question that God accompanied me on this unsteady stretch of life, but I was impervious to his comfort. For all intents and purposes I was agnostic.

In my late twenties, as I started to heal the things that drove me, I also began a long process of opening my heart to the possibility that God might value my life. I found myself more and more in the company of others who had chosen a spiritual path. For the first time in years I felt an occasional desire to pick up the Bible. My life still had pitfalls and challenges, but I no longer felt alone. I began to trust again the God of my childhood and over a period of time experienced a spiritual conversion.

I use the word "conversion" reluctantly because it implies a dramatic event. Most conversions of the heart, however, are experienced in subtle ways. For me it began as a need to surrender my destiny to something wiser than myself. I didn't hear a voice or see a vision, but I did experience a sense of relief.

It began when I realized I wasn't in control of my life. For a long, long time I'd resisted the idea of surrendering any part of my life as something weak and faulty, certainly not for someone with my lofty aspirations. But I kept finding myself in destructive situations of my own making. I'd have a unique opportunity, like making an exercise video or doing TV work, but it never lived up to my high expectations.

One day my efforts to force things to happen blew up in my face. In a single afternoon I managed to alienate an important media contact and seriously undermine my professional credibility. This humbling experience helped me see that my attempts to dictate my own destiny without any guidance from God, were as futile as trying to break down a brick wall by constantly flinging my body against it.

A few weeks later, as I scurried about the house trying to do my usual three things at once, I again experienced God's presence. I had a sudden sense of being directed into the living room from the kitchen where I was trying to make dinner, return phone calls, and finish my workout. So I turned off the stove, hung up the phone, put down the weights, and sat down on the sofa. There on the coffee table in front of me was the Bible I'd pulled out to read several weeks earlier. Of course in the days since I'd barely opened it once. Now I sat for a few minutes, feeling led on purpose, then picked up the Bible to read some Scripture (although I couldn't tell you today which verses). In all my busyness, I felt God remind me that I could turn my life over to his guidance, instead of relying so much on my own unsteady will power. It suddenly struck me how pointless it was to travel life's path any other way.

I sat there for a long time.

When I got up to return to my tasks, it was with a sense of peace. I understood in a way I'd never fully grasped before that I was born to participate in a relationship with God. For the first time ever I acknowledged my need for personal redemption.

I realized my approach to career, success, and life in general had been inherently misguided. These things were never supposed to be all about me, my fame, or fortune. Whatever gifts I'd been given as a creative person were a reflection of God. Surrendering my life to Christ wasn't a humiliating sign of weakness, but of freedom. I could look to, listen to, and lean upon someone bigger, and more in control, than me or any person.

Today as I continue my journey and invariably stumble, I fall into grace instead of an ever deepening pit. I've learned to rest in God's love, trust his plan, and practice my faith.

———✺———

There is guidance for each of us, and by lowly listening,
we shall hear the right word.
RALPH WALDO EMERSON

The combination of human nature and popular culture fosters the illusion that the things you do, money you earn, and the material things you accumulate are more pressing than the time you spend in prayer.

I labored under this misconception for years, and even today, knowing better, still drift into spiritual laziness. Sometimes I wish I could be transported to my grandparents' simple time, which revolved around family, church, and community. Prayer, reading, from the Bible, worship of God—these things came as naturally as breathing. But in today's fast-paced and morally ambivalent times, it takes an effort to connect with God through prayer. Despite my best intentions, I can frequently get to the end of a day and realize I haven't thought about God one time. The truth is there will never be a better time to make that effort than the present. I can't wait for life to be less complicated in order to honor my spirit.

In this respect, prayer is a lot like exercise. You can choose the plan, buy the equipment, and put on the workout gear, but at some point you have to start moving your body in order to get exercise. Fortunately, there's no right or wrong way to begin praying. God's available as soon as you turn your heart and mind to him.

As much as I love my grandiose retreats into the woods for time alone with God, I finally gave myself permission to implement brief moments of silence and prayer throughout the day. From the time I wake up in the morning to the moment my head hits the pillow at night, I try to have an ongoing dialogue with God. First thing in the morning, I thank him for the promise of a new day. Before I leave for work, even if it's sitting in the car before backing out of the driveway, I take a moment to appreciate the beauty of my surroundings and ask for guidance through the day ahead. When I go into a professional situation, like a speaking engagement or musical performance, I pray for wisdom in what I say and for the freedom to express feelings through music without an attack of nerves.

At the end of the day, about an hour before bedtime, I walk my dogs around the backyard and share my day with God. This is by far my best prayer time. Looking up at the evening sky never fails to move my heart with childlike awe at the mystery of God. My praying begins here, acknowledging the unfathomable gift of creation, and how grateful I am to be alive and witnessing it. Then I start in on my day, what went well (thank you!) and what didn't (help!). My prayer continues for people I know, the people I don't, and world events that have shaken or inspired me. Than I look around our scraggily backyard, worn down by the paws of my beloved and many dogs. I see the lights shining through the sliding glass windows of our simple, one-story home's den, where my husband sits watching TV. I give thanks then for everything I can think of in my life.

This helps me address the challenge of our times—the discontent I feel when I lose perspective of how very fortunate I really am.

You could pray without ceasing by just giving thanks for your many blessings. Thanking God for the simplest things in life—a hot meal, a warm bed at night, the health and safety of those near and dear to you—is a wonderful way to begin a prayer.

Throughout my lurching spiritual journey the gift of grace has moved me most of all. I feel the Father acknowledge and forgive my human failings in the same breath. Coming before God with a genuine willingness to listen and with the faith that he loves me beyond measure, is one of the most important actions I take in the course of a day. When my prayer time falls by the wayside, I immediately feel the spiritual deficit in my life.

197

Prayer nourishes the soul as tangibly as food and water nourish the body. It took many years trying to fix up my life from the outside for me to understand this. If you're serious about your quest for living the good life and realizing your potential for strength, balance, and inner beauty, you must honor your spiritual needs too. This is essential for respecting the whole person, because at some point in life you'll experience the presence of evil in the world and the dark side of human nature. These things are proven daily and are sure to challenge your faith. But what human nature sinks to is exactly what the human spirit can transcend. God is with you and me, in the quiet of a church, in the beauty of Creation, in selfless acts of kindness, and in his compassion for the human condition. He faithfully waits for us to loosen our grip on this world, to reach out for him and find him.

From one man he made every nation of men, that they should inhabit the whole earth; and he determined the times set for them and the exact places where they should live. God did this so that men would seek him and perhaps reach out for him and find him, though he is not far from each one of us. 'For in him we live and move and have our being.' As some of your own poets have said, 'We are his offspring.'

ACTS 17:26-28

The Power of Choice

Things you can do every day to impact your well-being

- **Remember a tranquil environment encourages a tranquil mind and can be a spiritual lifeline to God.** Even though you can pray in the middle of a traffic jam, there's something special about the sanctuary of a church, a garden, or a quiet corner of the house. Do you have a place to go, a retreat where you can commune with God?

- **Avoid things that spiritually demean.** I'm not suggesting you stick your head in the sand, but your soul is not well served by the tawdriness that overruns popular culture. If you're offended by a program on television, turn it off. Don't pick up magazines that exploit and then demean women. Instead seek out forms of art and entertainment that thrill your soul and lift your intelligence.

- **Think of what can you build into your life to stimulate spiritual growth.** Although your relationship to God is ultimately very personal, you need the fellowship of others who share your beliefs as a powerful incentive. When I felt my heart open to God, I sought the company of a dear woman for weekly Bible study. A simple request for guidance turned into a profound period of spiritual enlightenment. You can look to others for support and insight into your spiritual development, just as you do for help in other parts of your life like finances and health.

- **Write out for yourself some ways you can consistently incorporate your spiritual beliefs into your daily behavior.** You're a human

199

being with inevitable human failings, but a life of integrity reflects your spiritual beliefs as much as possible.

- **Live in the light of your own faith as the most powerful way to shed light on it.** As I've had the privilege to know and love people from all religious backgrounds and walks of life (people who have made my life better), I've always thought the best way to show respect for my own Christian faith is to be respectful of others. While I'd wish for anyone to know Jesus Christ as Savior, remember the spiritual path is ultimately a personal one.

- **Find support and inspiration in the insights of writers who have given their lives to God and the study of the Word.** I've found the writings of Max Lucado, Kathleen Norris, and C. S. Lewis to be enlightening and uplifting. I highly recommend *Celebration of Discipline, The Path to Spiritual Growth* by Richard J. Foster as a classic guide for the inward spiritual journey. Mr. Foster presents timeless, practical disciplines that encourage a closer walk with God and freedom from the trappings of our unsettling times.

Epilogue

*God is glorified in the fruitage
of our lives.*

JOEL S. GOLDSMITH

In 1944, after thirty years of a happy but grueling life in the country, Grandma and Grandpa Huber sold their farm and moved to a small, comfortable house in nearby Menomonie, Wisconsin. They continued to live active and fulfilling lives, which included social gatherings and travel they'd not had time for during the farming years. Grandpa spent many hours in his wood-shop, crafting handsome pieces of furniture that remain in our family today; Grandma created a beautiful rock garden behind the house and devoted more time to her fine seamstressing and crochet work. Together they maintained a sizeable vegetable garden and long rows of berry bushes in the backyard.

As they approached their sixties, my grandparents enjoyed town life. It was somewhat of a relief to no longer shoulder all the responsibilities of running a farm. Grandpa had time for more fishing, and Grandma was free to cultivate the flowering plants she loved so much. Still, my grandparents didn't deviate from the disciplined lifestyle they'd embraced on the farm. They continued to eat the harvest of their own garden, stayed active in and around the house, and got lots of natural exercise. The simplicity and spiritual focus of their daily lives remained much the same too.

I spent many summer vacations in Wisconsin, visiting Grandma Huber after Grandpa had passed away. The house in Menomonie was a child's delight, filled with violets and lace doilies and a curiosity down in the basement: an old wringer washing machine Grandma still used to wring out the water from the laundry she'd then hang to dry on the clothesline. The kitchen had a wonderful smell of old flour sacks, bacon grease, and spices that permeated the downstairs. The backyard still had a small vegetable garden with corn, tomatoes, and snap beans that our family enjoyed at the dinner table almost every evening. Berry bushes were heavy with ripe, delicious raspberries that were easy to pick and pop in the mouth.

The best part of Grandma Huber's house, though, was the rock garden out back—complete with a tiny, shallow pool right in the middle. Surrounded by mossy green grass, beautiful stones, and lilies of the valley, this was a magical place to sit and be still. I'd crouch beside that sweet pool and dangle my fingers in the water, scrunch my toes into the mossy grass, and feel utterly content.

I was enthralled by the simplicity and wholeness of my grandmother's life. I could not have realized this as a child, but I was responding to the timeless principles of the good life that had been the cornerstone of my grandparents' fruitful lives.

∞∞∞

The year I started to write this book, a package arrived in the mail from my mother. I opened it and carefully unwrapped the tissue paper from Grandma Huber's wedding dress. My mother had sent the dress, along with my grandparents' wedding picture, to see if I wanted to wear it for my own wedding.

The gift arrived at a perfect time. I'd been struggling with how to put into words what my personal life and professional experience had taught me about wellness. As I spread out that delicate, handmade wedding gown and gazed at the beautiful portrait of my grandparents as young newlyweds, I instinctively knew the book I had to write. It had to reflect simplicity and common sense. It had to resonate with a quest for health more than a search for the perfect body. I had to be honest about the arduous nature of my own path.

The sturdy stitches in my grandmother's wedding dress reminded me of the enduring principles by which my grandparents lived. Grandpa and Grandma innately understood what's taken me years to figure out: Life is precious and sometimes hard. Every day brings its share of work, joy, and sorrow. There's nothing more important than family and good friends. Human beings are designed to be physically active and live close to the land. Nature provides us with the best food we can eat. Simplicity is a timeless principle for good health and a good life. Quiet and rest are essential for the human spirit. Living in a steadfast relationship with God is the ultimate goal.

It's been years since I played in the rock garden behind Grandma Huber's house. Her teacups rest on the bureau in my living room, and her exquisite crochet work adorns pillow cases and lace-edged handkerchiefs scattered about the house. The picture of my grandparents' wedding day hangs on the wall as a mute reminder of the vibrant lives they once lived. It's also a testament to the temporal nature of this life.

When I gaze at that photograph, taken in 1913, I'm mindful of my own mortality and how passionately I want to reach age 90 in good health, with a sound mind. This is ultimately what our quest for wellness boils down to: How well can I live each day I'm given on this earth? What can I do on a daily basis to enhance my personal well-being? What simple, practical choices can I make to get the most out of life? How can I discover the strength, balance, and beauty within myself, and in doing so, honor God?

I hope this book has provided you with some answers to these questions, and that you're on your way to finding your truest and healthiest self. Trust your own wisdom and God's guidance. Celebrate daily your unique and remarkable qualities. Treat yourself kindly by refusing to draw comparisons to the appearance and accomplishments of others. Be gentle with your goals. Perfection will always be a tempting premise, but the imperfect process of life is the essence of life. In the end the heart-rending, breathtaking experience of life is your most precious birthright.

"It doesn't happen all at once . . . you become. It takes a long time."
MARGERY WILLIAMS IN *THE VELVETEEN RABBIT*

References

Batmanghelidj, F., M.D. *Your Body's Many Cries for Water.* Falls Church, Va.: Global Health Solutions. Excerpt used by permission.

Beattie, Melody. *Codependent No More.* Center City, Minn.: Hazelden Educational Materials, 1987, 1992.

Bennett, William J. *The Book of Virtues.* New York: Simon & Schuster, 1993. Excerpt used by permission.

Bringle, Mary Louise. "Confessions of a Glutton" *The Christian Century,* Oct. 25, 1989. Excerpt reprinted by permission from Christian Century Foundation.

Cooper, Dr. Kenneth H. *It's Better to Believe.* Nashville: Thomas Nelson, 1995.

Donnelly, Joseph E. *Living Anatomy.* Champaign, Ill.: Human Kinetics Books, 1990, 1982.

Gaesser, Glenn A. and Karin Kratina. *Eating Well, Living Well: When You Can't Diet Anymore.* Parker, Co.: Wheat Foods Council, 2000.

Frähm, David and Anne Frähm. *Healthy Habits, 20 Simple Ways to Improve Your Health.* Colorado Springs, Co.: Pinion Press, 1993.

Hemfelt, Dr. Robert, Dr. Frank Minirth, Dr. Paul Meier, Dr. Deborah Newman, Dr. Brian Newman. *Love Is a Choice.* Nashville: Thomas Nelson, 1991.

Peck, M. Scott. *The Road Less Traveled.* New York: Simon & Schuster, 1978. Excerpt reprinted by permission of Simon & Schuster.

Travis, John W., Ryan, Regina Sara. *Wellness Workbook.* Berkeley, Calif.: Ten Speed Press, 1981, 1988.

USDA Food Guide Pyramid

Whitfield, Charles L. *Co-dependence, Healing the Human Condition.* Deerfield Beach, Fla.: Health Communications, Inc., 1991. Excerpt used by permission.

References

Wilder, Laura Ingalls *The Long Winter.* New York: HarperCollins, 1940. Copyright renewed 1968 by Roger L. MacBride. Excerpt used by permission of HarperCollins Publishers.

Williams, Margery. *The Velveteen Rabbit.* New York: Simon & Schuster, 1983. Excerpt reprinted with the permission of Simon & Schuster Books for Young Readers, an imprint of Simon & Schuster Children's Publishing Division.